SEGMENTAL SPINAL INSTRUMENTATION

EDUARDO R. LUQUE, M.D.
EDITOR

SLACK

Printed in the United States of America

Library of Congress Catalog Card Number: 83-050287

ISBN: 0-943432-10-3

Published by: SLACK Incorporated
6900 Grove Rd.
Thorofare, NJ 08086

Last digit is print number: 8 7 6 5 4 3 2 1

Dedication

To all the crooked children of the world
and to those who have chosen to heal them.

CONTENTS

CONTRIBUTORS

Editor:

Eduardo R. Luque, MD, Medical Director and Chief, Hospital Dr. German Diaz Lombardo, Mexico City, Mexico.

Contributors:

Ben L. Allen, Jr., MD, Professor of Surgery and Pediatrics, Director of Pediatric Orthopedics and Spine Surgery, Division of Orthopedic Surgery, University of Texas Medical Branch, Galveston, TX.

Gordon W.D. Armstrong, MD, FRCS(C), Clinical Professor, University of Ottawa, Ontario, Canada; Chief Orthopedic Surgeon, Ottawa Civic Hospital, Ottawa, Ontario, Canada.

Paul Broadstone, MD, Fellow, Spine Deformity and Acute Injury Center, Kosair-Children's Hospital, Louisville, KY.

Alfredo Cardoso, MD, Surgeon Shriners Hospital, Mexico City Unit, Mexico.

James J. Carollo, MS, Director of Bioengineering, Texas Scottish Rite Hospital for Crippled Children, Dallas, TX.

Nelson Cassis, MD, FACS, Assistant Chief of Staff, Hospital Dr. German Diaz Lombardo, Mexico City, Mexico.

Francis Denis, MD, FRCS(C), FACS, Assistant Professor of Orthopedic Surgery, University of Minnesota; Chief of Spine Service, St. Paul-Ramsey Medical Center, St. Paul, MN; Attending Staff on Spine Service, Gillette Children's Hospital, St. Paul, MN; Spine Consultant, Veterans Hospital, Minneapolis, MN.

Ron L. Ferguson, MD, Associate Professor of Surgery and Pediatrics, Associate Director of Pediatric Orthopedic and Spine Surgery, Division of Orthopedic Surgery, University of Texas Medical Branch, Galveston, TX.

Charles F. Heinig, MD, Miller Clinic, Charlotte, NC; Department of Orthopedic Surgery, Charlotte Memorial Hospital, Charlotte, NC. Formerly, Chairman, Department of Orthopedic Surgery, Charlotte Memorial Hospital, Charlotte, NC.

John A. Herring, MD, Chief of Staff, Texas Scottish Rite Hospital for Crippled Children, Dallas, TX.

Richard T. Holt, MD, Clinical Instructor in Orthopedic Surgery, University of Louisville School of Medicine, Louisville, KY.

John R. Johnson, MD, Clinical Instructor in Orthopedic Surgery, University of Louisville School of Medicine, Louisville, KY.

Alfred Kahn III, MD, FACS, Assistant Clinical Professor of Orthopedic Surgery, University of Cincinnati, Cincinnati, OH; Director, Greater Cincinnati Spinal Deformity Center, Good Samaritan Hospital, Cincinnati, OH; Cincinnati Orthopedic Institute, Cincinnati, OH.

Andrew G.S. King, MB, ChB, FRACS, Associate Professor, Louisiania State University Medical Center, Department of Orthopedic Surgery, New Orleans, LA.

Kenton D. Leatherman, MD, Clinical Professor of the Department of Orthopedic Surgery, University of Louisville School of Medicine, Louisville, KY.

Rudolph F. Taddonio, MD, Clinical Associate Professor of Orthopedic Surgery, Director of the Scoliosis and Spinal Service, New York Medical College, Westchester County Medical Center, Valhalla, NY.

Dennis R. Wenger, MD, Assistant Chief of Staff, Texas Scottish Rite Hospital for Crippled Children; Associate Professor of Orthopedics, University of Texas Health Science Center, Dallas, TX.

State of the Art

1

Introduction

SEGMENTAL SPINAL INSTRUMENTATION WAS BORN of necessity in the treatment of severely paralyzed children with deformities of the spine. All the initial patients had an extremely low socioeconomic status and were therefore very difficult to see for repeated clinic visits over a prolonged period of time. Orthodox methods in vogue at the time gave miserable results.[6]

A chance observation in 1972 during a routine Harrington bar correction and arthrodesis led us to the conclusion that complete convex facetectomies would facilitate anteroposterior correction by distraction. Research at the Instituto Nacional de Antropologia in Mexico City provided the initial understanding of the segmental quality of the spine and of individual vertebral deformity, which explained our original chance observation.[7]

Many methods of individual vertebral fixation were studied, including the methods developed by Dr. Jacqueline Perry at Rancho Los Amigos and by Dr. Miguel Mendivil from Puebla, Mexico. Methyl methacrylate was used in conjunction with Knott rods or even Harrington bars for short segments. The real breakthrough in fixation of the spine, however, came from Dr. Javier Verdura. While

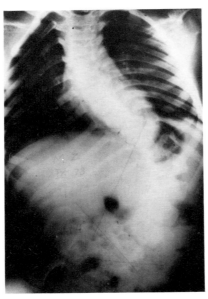

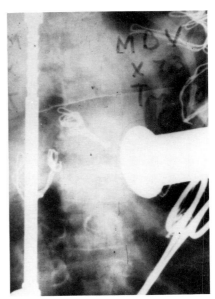

Fig. 1-1A. An 11-year-old girl with post-poliomyelitis sequelae, a 114° curve with severe pelvic obliquity (× 73).

B, Same patient after anterior diskectomies, posterior muscle release, and Hibbs-Risser arthrodesis (including complete facetectomies). Reduction is done by distraction (Harrington bar) and direct pressure over the apex (Risser localizer). Correction to −3° is obtained. Notice complete correction of rotational deformity and reversal of intervertebral spaces.

correcting a fracture-dislocation of the cervical spine, he showed us how to pass wires underneath the lamina.[16]

In 1973, correction of spinal deformity was recognized to have a direct relationship to bony deformity destruction and short soft-tissue elongation (Fig. 1-1). Fixation of the spine at that time consisted of Harrington bars with or without methyl methacrylate and one or two sublaminar wires (Fig. 1-2). Use of arthrodesis was determined based on an arbitrary knowledge of growth (Risser, Moe, and so forth) and on the psychosocial necessities of the patient.[8]

By 1974, it was obvious that segmental fixation had to correspond to segmental pathology. The addition of multiple points of fixation led to a distribution of forces.[8] By using either concave or convex Harrington rods, it became evident that distraction forces of correction occurred only in one plane. Transverse traction, pressure over the apex, and bringing the flexible ends over the convexity (Stainler, Cobb, Risser) gave maximum correction by wedging the intervertebral spaces at the apex, not at the flexible ends of the curve. Some derotation was done in structural curves, and pressure on growing epiphyses was changed in others.[4,6,12,14]

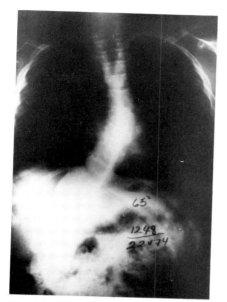

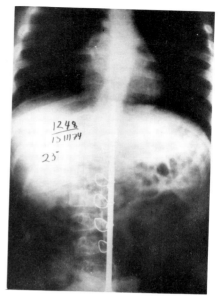

Fig. 1-2*A*. A 65° collapsing thoracolumbar curve with pelvic obliquity in a 10-year-old boy with post-poliomyelitis sequelae.

B to *D*, The same patient corrected to 23°. He has a level pelvis with a Harrington bar on the concave side, and segmental wires producing transverse traction. Notice that the intervertebral spaces are open at the apex. No correction of the rotational deformity was obtained.

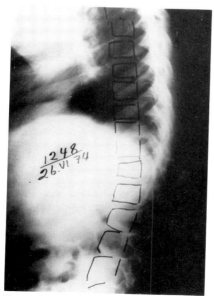

Fig. 1-2*C*.

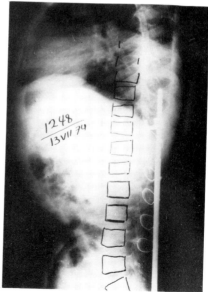

Fig. 1-2*D*.

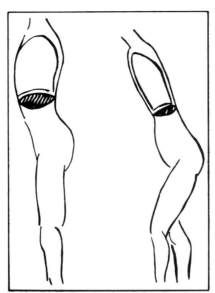

Fig. 1-3. Sagittal curves of the spine must be conserved. If the spine is flattened, ambulation will be hampered by the loss of lumbar lordosis. Flattening of the thoracic kyphosis brings about a loss of vital capacity.

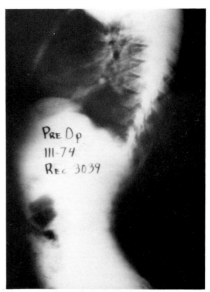

Fig. 1-4A. Lateral x-ray of a 10-year-old boy with post-poliomyelitis sequelae who has developed hyperlordosis in addition to a collapsing thoracolumbar scoliosis.

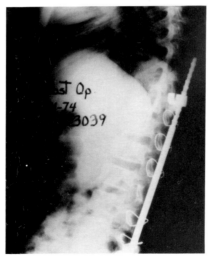

B, The same patient after Harrington concave bar distraction and transverse and posterior force correction with sublaminar wires, producing a flat lumbar back.

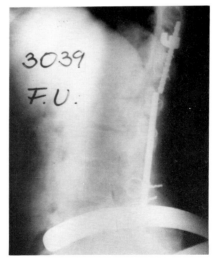

C, Same patient at the age of 13 yrs. Notice that an elongation of four teeth at the ratchet site has been done, and a posterior arthrodesis was attempted. The Harrington bar has broken at the first tooth of the ratchet, and pseudarthrosis is present at that point.

Further research using a three-dimensional computer model added to the basic anthropologic research findings about human posture and human anatomy.[3] It was realized that the teachings of this century—that a straight spine was a good spine—were wrong.[2,13,14] Physiologic curves served a purpose: better pulmonary ventilation and upright deambulation (Fig. 1-3). In other words, straight rodding of the lumbar and thoracolumbar spine had constituted two decades of iatrogenesis.

Basically, the problems of directing growth in a deformed spine, correction of average spine deformities, and internal fixation of the spine were evolutionized by 1975, but there were no follow-ups.[8] What we considered then to be major mistakes (mainly instrumentation failures) were really natural consequences of our available technology and progressing research (Fig. 1-4). Double rods (one concave and one convex), segmental sublaminar wiring, a sharp-angle derotational lever, and rods prebent to conform to a three-dimensional (anterior-posterior, sagittal, and axial) curve were the consequence. The formation of compensatory curves to produce an accepted residual deformity and the creation or correction of physiologic sagittal curves transformed our thinking about spine surgery (Fig. 1-5).

Many people were involved in this process, some of whom are mentioned in this text. Some are contributors to this book, but there are others who are no less important because of their enthusiasm and direct contributions. Surely to give a complete list of contributors is impossible.

What is SSI today? It is a tool, only as good as its craftsman. It has recognized individual vertebral pathology and three-dimensional deformities of the spine. Orthodox teachings about correction of bony deformities (transverse traction, eg, lateral bend, pressure on the apex, and so forth) and immobilization of one joint above and one joint below the deformity have been questioned. The physiologic importance of axial curves in producing adequate ambulation and progressive improvement in vital capacity has been studied. SSI is a basic support for the collapsing spine, be it the result of paralysis, tumor, infections, or spasms. It is also a corrective and supportive strut for low back disorders and other degenerative and destructive deformities.[11]

In growing children, we have considered the role of guiding spinal growth into a physiologic position, even after subperiosteal stripping (Fig. 1-6).

Owing to its supportive mechanics, SSI has become a tool in correcting and maintaining patients who for one reason or other cannot use external support.[1,5,15] Ultimately, it has served as a scaffold for the resection of entire segments of the spine, either to eradicate tumors or infections or to destroy enormous deformities and produce alignment (Fig. 1-7).[9]

SSI is still evolving and will keep on changing at an even greater pace than it has in the last decade. The basic principles will persist: individual vertebral pathology, destruction of bony deformity, lengthening of short soft-tissue structures, application of multiple forces of correction, shortening and complete alignment of the neural canal, individual vertebral fixation, maintaining sagittal physiologic curves, making a mechanical scaffold for structural defects of the bony vertebral column, and obtaining a balanced spine after correction. These principles are guiding us to a better method of immobilization and regulating growth in young

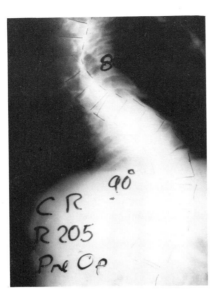

Fig. 1-5A. An 18-year-old patient with post-poliomyelitis sequelae with severe double major curves (thoracic 86°, lumbar 90°).

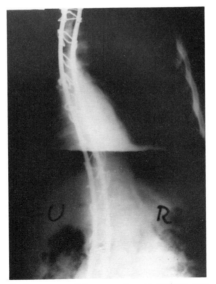

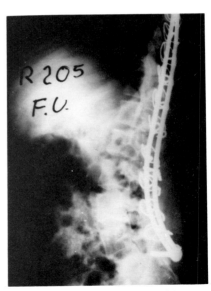

B, Seven-year follow-up of same patient, corrected with double-L rods covering the entire deformity, transverse traction pressure over the apex of the deformity, and alignment of the flexible ends of either curve. A Hibbs-Risser-type arthrodesis was done.

C, The lateral seven-year follow-up of the same patient showing the conservation of the lumbar lordosis and normal thoracic kyphosis.

children. New studies on physiologic axial curves and the way they change throughout the growing years are underway.

The one deformity in scoliosis that we have not corrected is apical rotation. By producing individual vertebral correction, we will someday control it both in young children and in adults. The complications and progress in our treatment are now unpredictable, however.

Correcting degenerative pathology of the spine has been barely considered up to now. It offers a great opportunity for improving the way of life of many of our patients. Spinal pathology that was once unsatisfactorily treated is now being treated successfully with SSI. Are we waiting too long, however? If we know that a spine is going to deform, can we not avoid it?

Many low back problems can be solved, some by distraction, some by producing lordosis, some simply by "holding" a correction. New knowledge of anatomy, pathology, and biomechanics will lead us to segmental treatment of many of these conditions. The advances in metallurgy and other fixating materials and methods will also give us increased capability to deal with spinal pathology, with unsuspected possibilities.

It would not be fair to finish this introduction without accepting that the road has been difficult; we have come across enormous amounts of problems and

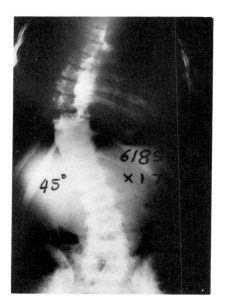
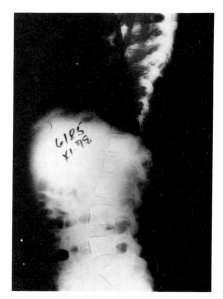

Fig. 1-6A and B. AP and lateral x-rays of a patient with idiopathic scoliosis of 45° on the AP view and a flat thoracic spine on the lateral. This is a female, age 9 yrs., with idiopathic scoliosis.

Fig. 1-6B.

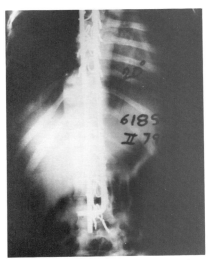

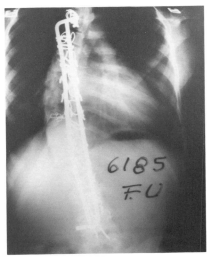

C, AP correction of the same patient to 20°. No arthrodesis was done.

D, Lateral x-ray of the same patient showing separation of the L bars caudally. No further correction was necessary. Notice maintenance of physiologic sagittal curves.

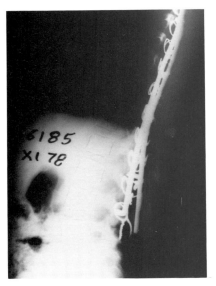

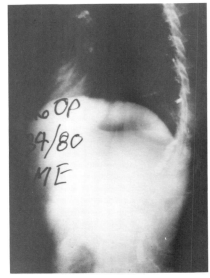

E, A three-year follow-up of same patient. She has lost correction, and her AP curve now measures 35°. She has grown 2.4 cm in the area of immobilization. She is still well balanced, has not used any external immobilization, and leads a normal life. No further surgery is programmed.

Fig. 1-7*A* and *B.* A 37-year-old man with a plasmocytema at the L1-T12 level. Myelographic study shows defect in the neural canal involving the corresponding vertebrae, with paraplegia.

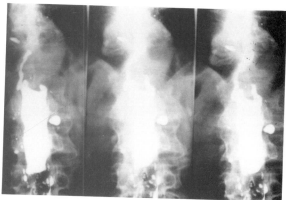

Fig. 1-7*B*.

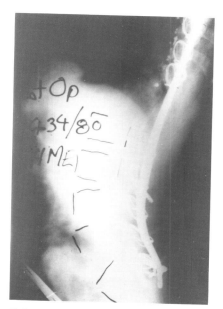

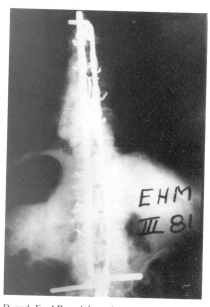

C, Lateral x-ray of same patient after total vertebrectomy of T12 and L1 in conjunction with tumor mass. His neurologic status was recovered.

D and *E*, AP and lateral x-rays of the same patient one year later after undergoing x-ray therapy and chemotherapy. Notice that there has been reconstitution of the anterior vertebral structures, with a collapse of one-half of the vertebral height. There is a solid fusion posteriorly. On last visit, this patient was neurologically normal and has never used external fixation.

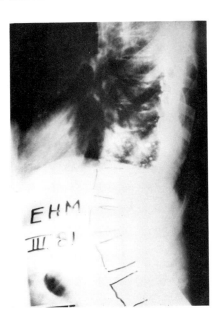

Fig. 1-7*E*.

complications as our technology and field of application have become greater. Correspondingly, we will find that our solutions are not infinite but like everything human, very much limited.

References

1. Allen BL, Ferguson RL: The Galveston technique for L rod instrumentation of the scoliotic spine. Symposium segmental spinal instrumentation. Spine 7(3):276-284, 1982.

2. Blount WP: Scoliosis and the Milwaukee brace. Hosp J Dis 19:152, 1958.

3. Chicurel UE, et al: Criterio Tridimensional en el Diagnostico de la Escoliosis. Memoria Sexto Congreso Academia Nacional de Ingenieria, pp 98-102, September, 1980.

4. Giannestras N: Personal communication.

5. Herring JA, Wenger DR: A preliminary report of 40 consecutive cases. Symposium segmental spinal instrumentation. Spine 7(3):285-298, 1982.

6. Luque ER: Anatomy of scoliosis and its correction. Clin Ortho 105:298, Nov-Dec, 1974.

7. Luque ER: Estudio Clinico Patologico de la Anatomia de la Escoliosis. Acta Ortopedica Latinoamericana. Vol. II, No. 2, p 182, August, 1975.

8. Luque ER: Paralytic scoliosis in growing children. Clin Ortho 163:202-209, March, 1982.

9. Luque ER: Vertebral column transposition. Ortho Trans 7:29, Spring, 1983.

10. Luque ER: Segmental spinal instrumentation for correction of scoliosis. Clin Ortho 163:192, March, 1982.

11. Luque ER: Surgical immobilization of the spine in elderly patients. Clin Ortho 273, June, 1978.

12. Risser JC, Norquist DM, Craig WA: Three types of body casts. Amer Acad Ortho Surgeons 10:131, 1953.

13. Risser JC: The application of body casts for the correction of scoliosis. Am Acad Ortho Surgeons 12:255, 1955.

14. Steindler A: Development and course of scoliosis, its mechanogenesis. Ortho Seminar Notes Vol. 1, Sect A, pp 39-43, 1950.

15. Sullivan JA, Conner SB: Comparison of Harrington instrumentation and segmental spinal instrumentation in the management of neuromuscular spinal deformity. Symposium segmental spinal instrumentation. Spine 7(3):299-304, 1982.

16. Verdura J: Personal communication.

Tailoring Surgery to Spinal Pathology

2

ALL TOO OFTEN WE AS surgeons sit down after a procedure and dictate an operative note, as if we had lifted a page out of a cookbook. The operation was "segmental spine instrumentation with fusion, D5 to L2, with right iliac crest graft." There is a need to classify procedures for insurance companies and coding and teaching purposes, but we must not lose sight of the fact that similar deformities may require different surgical approaches. The surgeon must evaluate the flexibility or the correctability of the curve and must always remember that balance is essential. We must strive for a compensated spine with as much flexibility left above and below the fused segment as possible.

Often, the spinal surgeon speaks about "correction" and "stabilization" of the spinal deformity. We speak of "fusing the deformity in situ" and have developed in our minds the concept that if we add more living bone or more inert metal to the deformed spine, we are going to "stabilize this deformity." Fusion of the spine will not hold back the advances of time and its effects on the spine. We must remember that unless we destroy or alter favorably the deforming forces or process, simply adding more bone or metal, at best, may retard the deformity. We also must remember that what we put in today, we will have to take out tomorrow. This may not be comforting to the surgeon. However, if we have enhanced the quality of life of a patient for years, we should not feel that we have failed. The internist has always been pleased with his efforts to prolong the life of his cardiac patient, even though the odds are that his luck will eventually run out.

Admittedly, with billions of people in the world, there are many problems that are similar. There are many cases in which fusion in situ is time proven, such as in spondylolisthesis where the slip angle is within normal limits and spinal alignment can be maintained by simply fusing L4 and L5 to the sacrum. Another patient with a similar amount of vertebral body displacement but a markedly increased slip angle may present with increased lordosis and altered body mechanics. To fuse this patient in situ and expect the same long-term good results is wishful thinking. The surgeon cannot cure everything. His motto must be to "do no harm."

The spinal surgeon must understand what he can accomplish with casts and orthoses in the treatment of acute and chronic spinal deformities. An orthosis on an older patient with severe deformity may not alter the x-ray results very much but may relieve the patient's pain considerably.

Development of S.S.I.

With this as our background, we must remember that it is not enough simply to quote the literature. We must be able to separate known facts from conjectures and impressions that surgeons may have. One must be objective and question the works and conclusions of ourselves, our associates, and the reports in the literature.

In the development of SSI, we must remember that progress is a result of successes, mistakes, and course corrections, just as in navigation.

Our editor, Dr. Luque, started off with building blocks of knowledge acquired during his life. They were honed into shape by many people with whom he came into contact, not the least, the late Dr. Joseph Risser. Dr. Harrington contributed further to his basic knowledge of spinal instrumentation. Knowing that certain cervical fractures could be held by sublaminar wires, the next step was the scientific marriage of sublaminar wires to Harrington rods, and thus the Harry-Lukes were born. This has now become a fairly well-established principle and concept in the orthopedist's mind. Further course corrections have been made to strengthen the system and remove the sometimes undesirable concept of correction of spinal deformity by distraction, and to strive for the ultimate: to rid the patient of postoperative casts and orthoses.

The smooth straight rod used in SSI migrated along the spine, just as it did in the clavicle or when placed across joints in fracture treatment. One of the first improvements was to put a bend in the end of the rod to form an "L." It was felt that this would permit the rod to be anchored securely to the spine by sublaminar wires, and if these two parallel L rods were lashed together, stability would result. It definitely was improved by these measures. It certainly helped reduce rod migration and had the desired property of allowing the young child's spine to grow as the upper L grew away from the lower L. On the other hand, if one had a tumor, infection, or fracture, further compression might have resulted as the rod settled and the L's approached each other. All of us can show examples of undesirable settling, and occasionally bone did bulge back into the canal and progressive neurologic deficits were noted. To overcome this undesirable effect, Dr. Luque placed a second L on both ends of the rod to create a C. This was a further improvement, but it still permitted rods with compound curves to rotate.

Further discussions with manufacturers brought about the concept of the closed-loop Luque rod of ³⁄₁₆″ and ¼″ diameter. Each rod would be bent with double 90-degree angles, and the parallel portions would be approximately two centimeters apart and securely welded together. This stopped the migration of one rod by the other, reduced rotation, and gave increased rigidity to the system, but at the expense of losing some of the desirable properties. The manufacturer and hospitals had to stock many lengths. Compound, complex bends could not be added to these rectangles. All one could add to this system were dorsal kyphosis and lumbar lordosis, since the rod could be bent only in one plane. Having the length established would prevent settling, but it also prevented growth from occurring. Thus, these closed rectangles had very limited use in scoliosis.

Many segmental spinal surgeons are now using a U-shaped rod, which is presently made from 60-centimeter L rods or specially obtained 120-centimeter

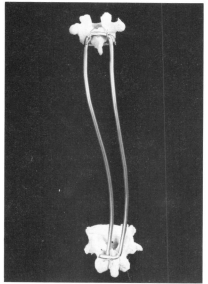

Fig. 2-1. The closed-loop Luque system with the rod fixed at either end to a vertebral specimen.

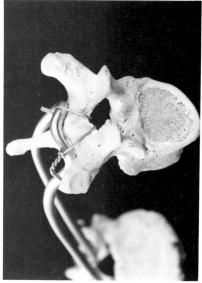

Fig. 2-2. A close-up of the contoured transverse portion of the rod as it is fixed and contoured to the lamina.

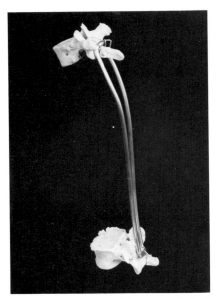 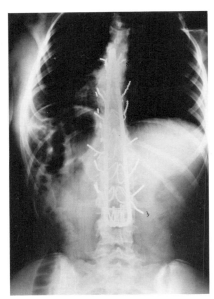

Fig. 2-3. A lateral view of these two rods fixed to vertebral body specimens, showing their compound bends.

Fig. 2-4. A U-shaped rod, which will allow for growth or settling to detour migration.

³⁄₁₆″ and ¼″ smooth rods. These can be contoured to give two right angles at the top or bottom of the U, which allows the parallel portions of the rods to be approximately two centimeters apart (Fig. 2-1). These may be further shaped across the U to contour to the lamina (Fig. 2-2). The parallel portions, because they have "free ends," can be contoured into lordosis and kyphosis, as well as complimentary complex scoliotic curves (Fig. 2-3). Once the exact length has been determined from a template, the rod ends are cut and bent and contoured again to fit the lower lamina. By serially wiring the "closed" loop to the upper or lower end of the deformity, the spine is aligned. This configuration has the advantage of lowering inventory by simply providing two rod sizes, 120 centimeters long, which can be made into a closed loop or left as an open-end U if settling or growth is desired (Fig. 2-4).

Again, manufacturers are being approached to consider the use of smooth stainless steel rods of ⁷⁄₃₂″ which would not be as rigid and hard to contour as the ¼″ rod and yet would give the orthopedic surgeon a little more versatility in performing instrumentation of the spine. These could be partially precontoured by the manufacturer to allow for easy handling, storage, and autoclaving by hospitals.

It is obvious by now that not all of us agree on the ideal sizes and shapes of rods, or the number of sizes of wire to be used. One must remember that this is a new procedure that is in a state of evolution. A great part of the success of SSI rests not with the materials but with the surgeon's ability to use them. Rarely before has he been asked to bend metals at the operating table, other than to bend the sideplate a few degrees to fit around the bony deformity. Now we are presenting him with a tool that requires him to construct compound curves with complimentary curves parallel to each other and two centimeters apart throughout most of their course. It must be remembered that the spinal deformity and the contoured rod must fit when the deformity is corrected. One must also have a concept of biomechanics; certainly, the stresses exerted on a rod by a 100-pound person are not the same as in a 250-pound person. One does not need the same size rod in an active 30-year-old male as he does in a 70-year-old osteoporotic female.

Economically, it is to everyone's advantage to have two or three sizes of rods partially contoured by the manufacturer, which can be universally adapted to the majority of spinal problems. It reduces the high, costly inventory of implants that now make so many systems undesirable.

A great deal of work and thought have gone into the wires. Initially, they were taken off the spool with two raw cut ends, which could easily puncture surgical gloves and lead to contamination. Now many of us use double wires that are beaded at each end to facilitate passage. Others of us use single double-beaded 12-inch 16- or 18-gauge stainless steel wires, which obviate the problem of sharp ends on the wires during the entire procedure, since they do not need to be cut apart before they are tied.

One of the problems that concerns the author is that although "all men are created equal," many things happen to us during our maturation and development. Obviously, all surgeons do not possess the same motor skills or dexterity, nor do they all have the same ability to remain mentally alert for prolonged periods of time. The skills and mental alertness are paramount to the proper use of this method, since complications will result from the multiple sublaminar wires being untied during the procedure. Various methods have been devised to minimize the danger to the cord and roots. One must make an adequately sized opening in the interlaminar area so that the wire can be passed smoothly and easily. The wire should be either crimped, twisted, or secured about the lamina. Some have used small rubber tubes over the wire, much as one would place a clasp over a Western string tie.

It is essential that once the wires are tightened, they all be twisted in the same direction, preferably clockwise. Otherwise, chaos and confusion will develop as the wires are serially tightened while correction is being obtained. They should not be overtightened, and, basically, the wire twisting should be used to snug the rod in place once the team has approximated the rod to the lamina. It appears that at least six turns should be left on each wire when it is cut. The wire should be turned down so that each strand assumes a 45-degree inclination to the rod. It is essential that the cut ends be turned down, and they can be used to hold bone graft down in the gutters lateral to the rods. It is desirable to bind down the end wires to prevent them from popping up. Fusing one level above or below the rod may also be desirable at times in neuromuscular or osteoporotic individuals, in whom adding on is apt to occur naturally. Most authors agree that double wiring of the ends of the rods is sufficient. However, others doubly wire each level.

Although we wish to stress the use of SSI, we must remember that many are

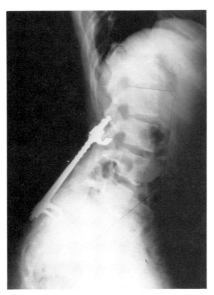

Fig. 2-5. The use of Harrington rods in the lumbar area, which demonstrates its extreme ability to flatten the spine.

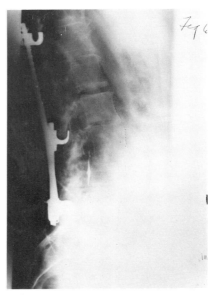

Figs. 2-6 and 2-7. Contoured Harrington rods with lordosis bent into them. Later, postoperatively, the longer rod has rotated into a kyphotic position.

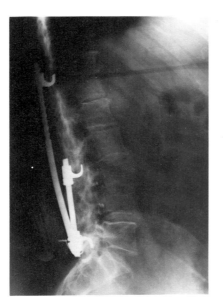

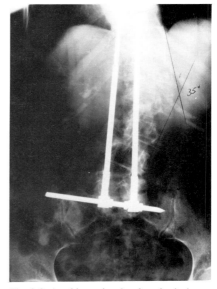

Fig. 2-8. An older patient in whom lordosis was reduced for a while until the transsacral bar was cut out and all correction was lost.

just now mastering the use of the somewhat simpler Harrington technique. We do not expect that everyone will discard that technique, even though we feel that SSI has many advantages. In the hands of many surgeons, Harrington instrumentation is the preferred treatment. It is possible to place the Harrington rod in its usual position, pass individual wires, and tie each as it is passed to reduce the hazards. We must remember that the Harrington system tends to flatten the normal curvatures, and that even when bent, it may rotate from a form of lordosis in the lumbar area to a kyphotic position, even when it has had sublaminar wiring (Figs. 2-5, 2-6, and 2-7). It would seem that Harry-Lukes are best placed above L3 to reduce the unpleasant deformity of flattening of the lumbosacral area. The use of the transsacral bar needs to be discarded for the same reason (Fig. 2-8). Above L2 in the deformed spine, there is not much room for sublaminar hook placement, since the cord tends to be displaced toward the concavity, where the lamina is foreshortened.

Often, wire placement on the convexity of the curve is given the credit for nerve root problems. The surgeon must pay attention to the fact that in scoliosis, the vertebrae are deformed. Thus, in their correction, one must remove the elongated lamina and superior facets on the convexity. As the spine is moved toward the concavity in the shortening procedures or with minimal distraction, the nerve roots are impaled against the pedicle by the elongated superior facets of the vertebra below it. In kyphosis, a similar situation may exist. In this case, the apical superior facets and lamina are elongated and curved forward. Extension may result in cord or nerve root compression.

Tumors

In years past, a patient with a malignancy of the spine did not present a major problem to the spinal surgeon because the problem was short-lived. Today, the spinal lesion patient may have his life expectancy altered markedly, so that now we have to recognize the fact that a collapsed vertebra at T12, for example, may be "sterilized" by high-energy treatment and chemotherapy. The oncologist then presents the orthopedic surgeon with a deformity in a partially paralyzed patient with a life expectancy that may be a matter of years. The oncologist wishes to have the spine "stabilized." The treatment often creates problems for the spinal surgeon, who on opening the spine finds that all the paravertebral muscles and ligaments are a fused mass of necrotic "bacon-like" material. The vertebrae appear like a sequestrum. At this time, metallic rod stabilization is often complicated by the fact that four weeks later, the wound is not healed. Thus, it is important to become part of the team and get in on the planning of treatment. If the orthopedist can get a two-week head start on the irradiation therapist or can get him to use

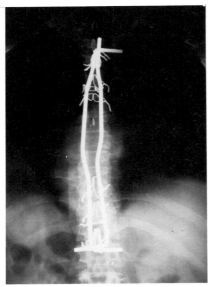 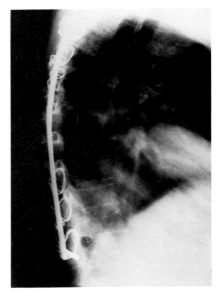

Figs. 2-9 and 2-10. A tumor patient who has had rods contoured to go around the decompressed areas, to put pressure over the pedicles of the transverse processes. This happens to be a case of metastatic lung cancer.

Fig. 2-10.

lateral ports, the healing problem may be avoided. Chemotherapy may also slow down healing of wounds in certain cases. If the tumor therapy team concept can be established and the sequence of therapy decided for the good of the patient, this will be an important first step.

The author's neurosurgical colleagues have recognized that decompressive laminectomy further destabilizes most tumor patients' spines. Thus, we combine our surgical efforts and stabilize with SSI as part of the initial therapy. One must know if there is more than one spinal lesion in the area. On one occasion, three areas of blockage in a prostate cancer patient were recognized and decompressed. Long rods were fashioned to span all the needed vertebrae. The sequence of surgery may be extremely important for the patient. The untreated hypernephroma is best stabilized and the rods best contoured lateral to the area to be decompressed (Figs. 2-9 and 2-10). Once the fixation is secured, the lid over the hypernephroma may be removed. These tumors are notorious as bleeders.

In the case of tumors such as lymphomas and myelomas, these people may live long periods of time. It is often surgically simple to remove much of these soft tumors and bony fragments from under the cord. One may wish to let the spine slowly settle down a U-shaped rod or perhaps to place methyl methacrylate in the anterior shell and maintain the height. It may be desirable to bone graft these people if it is felt that they have a life expectancy of more than six months.

The tumor patient is often the most appreciative individual in the surgeon's

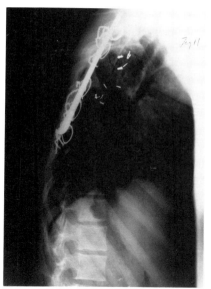 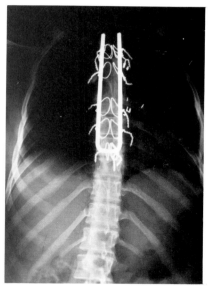

Figs. 2-11 and 2-12. A child with a giant cell tumor stabilized with a U-shaped Luque rod with anterior and posterior surgery. The U shape will permit growth or settling.

Fig. 2-12.

practice. He may not live many years, but the fact that he is not paralyzed and is comfortable is very important. The quantity of life is not as important to him as the quality. These patients routinely have told the author that once their spine was decompressed and stabilized, the pain relief they obtained from the surgery was unbelievable. It has reduced their need for narcotics, and many of those who were partially paralyzed have been able to return to ambulation and to maintain bladder and bowel control until the final insult.

Benign tumors of the spine may lead to instability. A giant cell tumor at D5 in a 14-year-old girl is a case in point. Excision of most of the body and posterior elements with SSI fixation and bone grafting posteriorly was followed a few days later by anterior body resection and bone grafting with ribs. Here, a U-shaped rod would allow for settling or growth (Figs. 2-11 and 2-12).

Neuromuscular Problems

SSI in patients with neuromuscular problems has been most rewarding. Whether the problem is due to polio, cerebral palsy, posttraumatic paralysis, meningomyeloceles, or other causes of collapsing spine, SSI offers an excellent

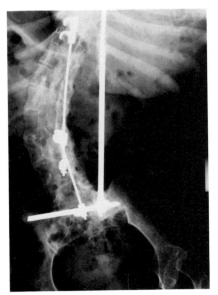
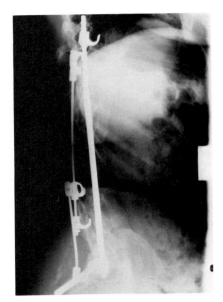

Figs. 2-13 and 2-14. Two x-rays of an old polio patient who had a transsacral rod placed 20 years before. The bar has dislocated, and the hooks and rod have migrated into the sacrum, necessitating removal because of pain in an S1 nerve root.

Fig. 2-14.

method of correction and fixation of the spine until fusion is complete. The Galveston technique is one method of anchoring the pelvis and holding the spine securely over the midline. These are difficult rods to contour, and it must be stressed that if they are poorly contoured, the correction will be poor. It may be necessary to perform multiple procedures on the severely deformed patient with pelvic obliquity before SSI is done. Then pelvic obliquity may be corrected and held by well-contoured rods.

We must remember that many disastrous results have been recorded from the use of alar hooks and transsacral bars, since they are easy to dislodge. In the paralyzed sitter, it appears desirable to increase his lordosis and place the weight on his thighs. The Harrington system flattens the spine and places the weight on the ischial tuberosities and the tip of the sacrum. Dr. Harrington recognized this undesirable side effect of lessening lordosis and, at times, put his hooks essentially upside-down on a transsacral bar (Figs. 2-13 and 2-14). He tried to get the rod as far forward in the spinal column as he could. In spite of this, the transsacral bars loosened, and the hooks would tend to migrate into the sacral canal, creating delayed problems.

The child with a meningomyelocele may present real problems of skin coverage. Here it is advisable to put one's rods out laterally away from the midline, where they can be covered by better tissues. The rods can be anchored to the

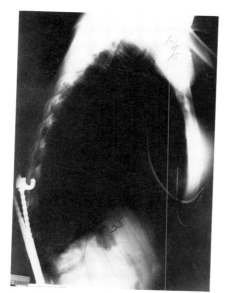

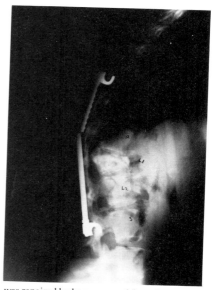

Figs. 2-15, 2-16, 2-17, and 2-18. A young lady who sustained a compression fracture and was felt to be neurologically complete. Thus, Harrington instrumentation was carried out. It was left unprotected. One rod moved out after six weeks and was removed. The second rod broke at seven months. The resulting pseudarthrosis was repaired by bone removal from the canal by the eggshell approach. The patient regained sensation and movement nine months after the third procedure. Obviously, she had an incomplete lesion that deserved a chance at bone removal. The final outcome is not known.

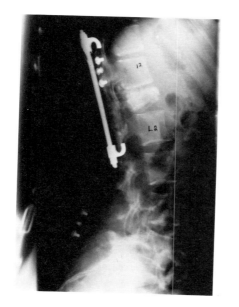

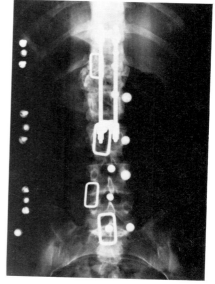

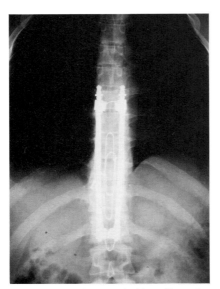

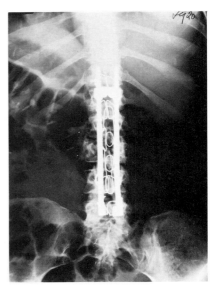

Fig. 2-19. A Harrington rod with ancillary wire fixation to limit excursion of the spine and, hence, reduce rod cut out. Ancillary orthosis should be used.

Fig. 2-20. Contoured Harrington rods with sublaminar wire fixation, which lessens rod breakage and displacement and may not require external immobilization.

pedicles or around the congenitally fused segments. Excellent fixation with the Galveston technique has been used by the author.

Fractures

In general, most orthopedists and neurosurgeons feel that early stabilization of spinal fractures and fracture-dislocations is advisable. A spinal cord injury is a disaster for the individual and his community. Anything that can be done to lessen the impact is desirable. It is essential to remove bone from the canal no matter what method is used. Stabilization of the spinal fracture or fracture-dislocation is not for all orthopedic surgeons. The treatment must depend on the facilities that are available and the skill of the surgeon. Today, rapid transportation is available to most people.

Many people believe that it is a simple matter to place two Harrington rods parallel to one another, with the upper hook two levels above the unstable motion segment and the lower hooks two segments below it. This does not lead to stable fixation. Many spines have been overdistracted. Fragments do not automatically just pop back into place upon distraction. External immobilization is necessary, because the rod will pop out of place or break (Figs. 2-15 to 2-18). The use of ancillary wire fixation may limit the excursion (Fig. 2-19). Sublaminar wires may also help (Fig. 2-20). The method is best applied when the lower hook is placed between L1 and L3, or if the lower hook is placed at L4, the fusion is to L3 or above, and the rod is to be removed 18 to 24 months later.

SSI can provide stability and maintain distraction if a closed-loop system is utilized and is especially desirable when a fixation extends to the lower cervical and upper dorsal spine (Figs. 2-21 and 2-22). The double L rod will allow for settling, but in the complete lesion, this probably makes no difference. However, on three occasions, lesions described as complete by others who had removed bone from the canals have shown neurologic improvement. It is hard to determine exactly what is going on in the multiply injured individual, especially with a closed head injury. The patient should be given every chance. The bone should be removed from the canal. He cannot be hurt if he is neurologically complete. If one is careful, the patient might be helped.

When it is desirable to fix lower vertebral body fractures, such as L4 and L5, SSI involving the ala or wings of the ilium can provide a secure anchor. It allows for maintenance of lordosis and removes the need for pantaloon casts. This same method may be used to hold or partially reduce spondylolisthesis deformities.

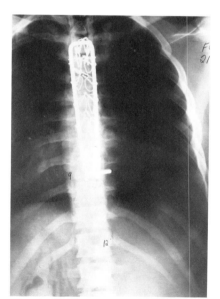

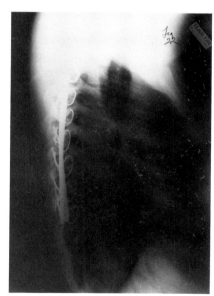

Figs. 2-21 and 2-22. A contoured closed-loop Luque rod, which provides excellent fixation and alignment of this D6 fracture-dislocation.

Fig. 2-22.

The question that still exists in the minds of many is, "How long do you fuse the spine?" In the neurologically intact individual, probably the least number of vertebrae that will prevent recurrence of the deformity should be fused. In the neurologically complete individual, fusion to the sacrum and three levels above the lesion probably is a good starting rule. The use of SSI in the growing child should be considered for the deformity that cannot be controlled by orthosis or if a fusion may not be desirable. Periosteal stripping does not prevent spinal growth. This has been shown by Dr. Luque repeatedly.

In our area, people used to feel that the deformity should be permitted to grow until maturity, and once it was "ripe," if it was bad enough, should be corrected. Fortunately, the natural history approach is no longer widely practiced. It is much easier to correct simple deformities, even if more than one operation is required. Simply resecting many vertebrae in the severely kyphotic child with a neuromuscular disorder may help correct the gibbus but will not leave room for growth of abdominal contents. Thus, if by the use of internal splinting of these children with insensitive skins, we could grow the spine straighter, we could reduce a lot of agony for the patient and surgeon.

There are other congenital problems, such as hemivertebra, that might be managed by simple excision and sublaminar wiring to rods bent in the corrected position.

There has been some enthusiasm for using SSI in persons who appear headed for disastrous deformity with ankylosing spondylitis. It would seem reasonable to try to prevent the loss of lumbar lordosis and minimize the excessive dorsal kyphosis. These spines might simply ankylose themselves and maintain relatively normal statures. The dura is extremely thin, and it might be advisable to do intralaminar wiring or wiring through the bases of the spinous processes. Recently, while doing a one-stage osteotomy and partial vertebrectomy (Eggshell Procedure), we were unable, clinically or in the laboratory, to find any tissue around the cord that could be identified as dura. On occasion, the ligaments and dura appear to ossify completely. This should be kept in mind and the procedure tailored to address this problem.

Persons with osteoporosis may be significantly improved by SSI. At the present time, the author has operated on three persons whose kyphotic deformities progressed rapidly before age 55. In the first (a fireman), a set of L rods was used, and good correction was obtained. We slowly lost some of this as the rods tended to migrate apart and elongate. He has since been working two years and is happy with his result. In the two subsequent cases, closed-loop segmental spinal instrumentation was used (Figs. 2-23 to 2-25). In each case, multiple compression fractures had occurred in rapid succession. An osteoporotic work-up, including labeled bone biopsies, failed to find a cause. In both, the spines were corrected to within normal curvatures. While the fixation was being secured to the lamina, the previously fractured vertebrae were noted on x-ray examination to open up anteriorly. Thus, it was apparent that closed osteoclasis had occurred at multiple levels. Both these patients were markedly improved. One lady has returned to gainful employment as a schoolteacher. The other lady has returned to being a homemaker.

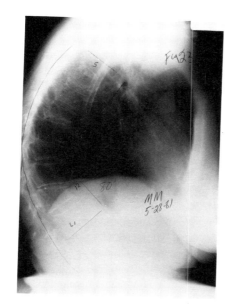

Figs. 2-23, 2-24, and 2-25. A 53-year-old lady who had acute fractures secondary to osteoporosis at D8, D10, and D12. She was unable to work prior to her surgery, and her curve had reached 80 degrees. It was corrected with closed-loop Luque rods to 36 degrees. Two years later, she is working as a schoolteacher. The curve is painless and has settled to 45 degrees.

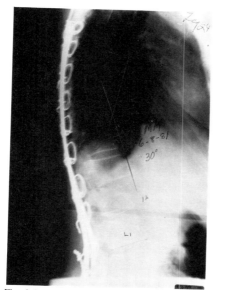

Fig. 2-24.

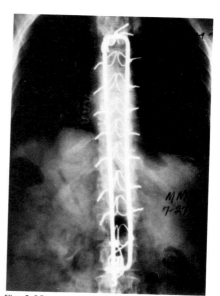

Fig. 2-25.

Certainly, this should not be done in every osteoporotic individual.

There are certain metabolic problems that befall younger people, such as deformities seen in persons taking large doses of cortisone for Crohn's disease or arthritis. Rarely, young people have idiopathic adolescent osteoporosis, and SSI might help these people. Another group of people who might be helped are those who develop extreme osteoporosis while on renal dialysis or after having kidney transplantation.

The patient with osteogenesis imperfecta and associated spinal deformity may also find benefit from SSI. Those of us who have operated on osteogenesis imperfecta patients with scoliosis in the past using Harrington rods have seen good initial correction melt away rapidly as the rods sink into the lamina. The addition of methyl methacrylate to the ends of the rods has helped some. The rod size must be matched to the patient's bones, for if the rods are too rigid, the pedicles may be simply elongated and the deformity may recur. An orthosis may be a desirable adjunct to the SSI in such a case, until the fusion is solid.

There are an increasing number of people who feel that if it is possible to have their deformities corrected surgically so that they do not have to wear casts, then they are willing to try this newer approach to their problem. Many of them remember as children being offered treatment with Risser turnbuckle casts and had instead decided to live with their deformities. As the deformities have progressed and arthritic symptoms have developed, they now would like to have some relief, but they still do not wish to use a cast.

There are persons who have skin afflictions, such as psoriasis, who would not tolerate casts well. Children with scoliosis and limb bud deficiencies cannot tolerate body jackets, since they need their body surfaces to control their body temperatures. Also, there are those people who cannot consider surgery emotionally if they are going to be incarcerated in a cast or brace. Persons with severe curves and respiratory problems can also be managed with SSI better than with previously available methods.

Techniques that shorten the spine are getting more attention. The Dwyer and Zielke methods shorten the spine by disk and end-plate resection; some shortening will occur. The disadvantage of these procedures is that they are frequently coupled with the need for a secondary posterior approach. The situation that bothers some of us is that these procedures strip away several segmental vertebral vessels at the apices of these curves. With a second posterior operation, additional vessels are by necessity injured, thus further lessening the blood supply to the cord.

There are many factors that bring about paralysis during these procedures. However, it seems logical to preserve as many vessels as possible while correcting severe curves. Thus, Dr. Luque and the author feel that if it is possible to save the segmental vessels and still do vertebrectomies, this should be done. It is easy to remove the disk material anteriorly, and it is possible to remove the bodies at the apices subperiosteally. The resulting tube of periosteum can be stuffed with cancellous bone and ribs and the tube sutured, producing a relatively limber segment, usually five to seven vertebrae in length. The tube becomes flexible, like a hot dog. Postoperatively, tong-gravity traction or a Risser turnbuckle cast may be used to obtain correction, gradually stretching out the intercostal and abdominal muscles. Ten to fourteen days later, a posterior approach is carried out. During the second stage, multiple facetectomies and partial laminectomies may be performed, or if more correction is deemed necessary, the posterior elements of one or more vertebrae may be removed. It soon becomes apparent that four or more ribs on the concavity will need to be removed to let the spinal column move over. This permits derotation of the chest cavity and the spinal column. The spinal column is permitted to shorten, and correction will be maintained by segmental instrumentation. One must always remember not to correct the primary curve beyond the point that the compensatory curves can balance. For this spinal stabilization, a 120-centimeter rod may be fashioned into a U and contoured to fit the lamina. The desired scoliotic, kyphotic, and lordotic curves can be added. Once the desired length is established, the rod can be cut off and its lower end contoured. We have not used spinal cord monitoring but do use the wake-up test routinely.

An area that has not been mentioned in this chapter is the role of SSI in idiopathic scoliosis. The average scoliotic surgeon is not comfortable doing SSI for the simplest curves. However, we utilize SSI in our worst cases. Harrington instrumentation has fewer complications for most surgeons, but it is still the silent flattener of backs, which must be considered an undesirable sequela to the use of the straight distraction rod.

The 50- to 60-degree idiopathic curve probably is best treated by the average orthopedic surgeon using Harrington instrumentation. If he places the lower hook in the intralaminar rather than the sublaminar area and uses Moe square rods, he can build in some lordosis and kyphosis. If individual wires are then passed and tied sequentially, he may lessen his concern over paralysis. In general, we have found that approximately eight degrees of additional correction can be obtained after the wires are tightened. At this point, however, the author cautions the surgeon not to jack up his Harrington rod one or two more notches because the rod appears to have loosened. The natural instinct is to get a little more correction and take up the slack. This is how we believe many surgeons doing "Harry-Luke" procedures needlessly pick up neurologic deficits.

Harrington instrumentation has fallen short of what SSI can accomplish with severe scoliotic curves. SSI gives patients with severe chest deformities and respiratory problems stability without the need for casts and orthoses. Vertebral body resections, whether they are done as a one-stage Eggshell Procedure or by a two-stage transthoracic approach with multiple diskectomies and vertebrectomies, must be determined by the need for correction and by the surgeon's confidence and level of skill. There is little doubt that greater correction of spinal deformities can be accomplished by shortening of the spine than we have known by previous methods of distraction. We must remember that we can do this at the expense of losing abdominal and thoracic cavity space.

Editor's Commentary

Individualizing, projecting, and predicting have probably been brought out as surgical prerequisites more by SSI than by any other orthopedic technique in the past. More than ever, surgical judgment, a surgeon's individual ability, and hospital facilities play a very important part in the final outcome of the correction of spine deformity and immobilizing with SSI.

The concept that SSI is a finite procedure is of extreme importance, especially in degenerative diseases and in growing children. The realization that SSI is a changing tool that has allowed us to do things unthinkable ten years ago underlies the spirit of this book. New materials and new techniques to correct deformities are still ahead, together with their corresponding dangers and learning process.

Biomechanics of Segmental Spinal Instrumentation

3

Introduction

WHEN A PHYSICAL IMPAIRMENT such as scoliosis is defined in mechanical terms and then treated with mechanical methods, biomechanical analysis can provide valuable information regarding the effectiveness of treatment. This is not a unique concept, since prior studies of scoliosis have included biomechanical descriptions of treatment methods (Milwaukee brace, Harrington instrumentation, Dwyer anterior instrumentation, Weiss spring). In several of these studies, the desirability of transversely applied forces was suggested; however, only recently has surgical instrumentation capable of providing transverse forces been available.[2,4,6,9,14] Luque's method of segmental spinal instrumentation provides segmental correction and fixation by applying a transverse force at every vertebra, providing stability in the frontal, sagittal, and transverse planes.[2,4] In this chapter, we address the biomechanics of the Luque method of segmental spinal instrumen-

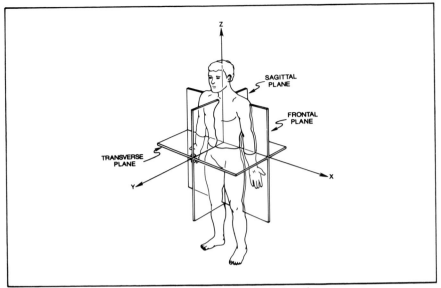

Fig. 3-1. Coordinate system to define anatomic planes and spinal motion.

tation (SSI) and compare its effectiveness with that of the Harrington distraction method. We begin by describing the mechanical principles underlying segmental instrumentation and then present the results of in vitro animal studies performed to evaluate these theoretical concepts.

Scoliosis as a Three-Dimensional Deformity

Although the clinician sometimes thinks of scoliosis as primarily a lateral curvature of the spine, the three-dimensional nature of the deformity cannot be overlooked. In most cases, lateral deformity is accompanied by a change in the normal sagittal plane contour, as well as axial rotation of the vertebrae near the apex of the curve. Because of this, a truly accurate mechanical analysis of methods of scoliosis correction requires a complex mathematical model.[1,5] Unfortunately, this type of representation offers little help to the clinician whose measure of scoliosis progression is in terms of a two-dimensional Cobb angle taken from a planar radiograph. Recognizing this problem, White and Panjabi suggested a simple two-dimensional model that described the response of an externally loaded spine in three mutually orthogonal planes, each evaluated independently.[14] Although this model did not consider the coupling effects commonly seen between planes (eg, axial rotation with lateral bending), it did agree with the basic trends that were seen in their three-dimensional mathematical model, in terms of model response to externally applied loads. Therefore, a simplistic model can be considered relatively accurate for qualitative comparison of correction techniques. The model used in this study is similar to White and Panjabi's, with additional segments included to evaluate the performance of a segmental approach such as Luque's.

For clinical purposes, spinal motion has traditionally been defined in reference to the three anatomic planes, that is, the frontal, sagittal, and transverse planes. At the intersection of these planes lie the three principle axes by which all three-dimensional motion is defined (X, Y, Z) (Fig. 3-1). For our purposes, we define the X axis as the intersection of the frontal and transverse planes, the Y axis as the intersection of the sagittal and transverse planes, and the Z axis as the intersection of the frontal and sagittal planes. The origin of the coordinate system is that point which is contained in all three planes, located roughly at the center of mass of the body. We refer to this coordinate system throughout the following discussion.

The Role of Instrumentation in Scoliosis Surgery

The primary goals of scoliosis surgery are curve correction and stabilization to avoid progressive deformity in adult life. By producing forces that counteract the scoliotic spine's inherent tendency to buckle, effective scoliosis instrumentation provides efficient correction and the early structural support required to insure formation of a solid fusion mass.[3]

Regardless of the means by which an instrumentation method applies corrective forces, correction and subsequent stabilization are affected by the production of bending moments at the intervertebral disks. This implies that the larger the bending moment produced, the greater the potential for curve correction, assuming constant rigidity in the spine. Therefore, one limiting factor in curve correction is the ultimate strength of the bone-metal interface. Biomechanical studies by Schultz and Hirsch have shown the importance of these concepts in distraction instrumentation.[7] These authors documented a correction limit where further distraction can neither be maintained without failure at the bone-metal interface nor produce any appreciable increase in the intervertebral bending moments. This phenomenon has also been documented clinically by Waugh and in the laboratory by Wenger et al.[11,13]

An obvious additional limiting factor in scoliosis correction is neurologic function, since excessive distraction forces may produce cord ischemia with neurologic sequelae.

Because the most effective system for obtaining and maintaining correction in scoliosis must produce the maximum corrective force without exceeding the ultimate strength of the bone-metal interface, each instrumentation method is evaluated in terms of its potential to: (1) produce corrective bending moments (Biomechanics of Correction), and (2) maintain the forces it produces without failure (Biomechanics of Failure).

Biomechanics of Correction

When a force is applied to a rigid body some distance from a specific axis, a twisting or rotational effect is produced about that axis. This effect is called a "moment of a force," or more simply a "moment." Since the applied force tends to deform the rigid body, the term "bending moment" is often employed.

A bending moment is a vector quantity and as such can be resolved into components that lie in each of the anatomic planes. The magnitude of each component is defined as the product of the force component in that plane times the perpendicular distance between the line of action of the force and an axis perpendicular to the plane. Therefore, bending moments about the X axis result from those force components that lie in the sagittal plane. Similarly, moments about the Y and Z axes are produced by force components in the frontal and transverse planes, respectively. This description is important because the following discussion of the biomechanics of correction is concerned with specifying which force components exist with each scoliosis instrumentation method.

Frontal Plane Correction

For a lateral curve in the frontal plane, corrective bending moments about the Y axis can be produced by applying longitudinal forces (axial distraction), transverse forces, or a combination of the two. With the Harrington method, the distraction rod produces a force whose major component is in the direction of the Z axis. Since the rod itself is oriented longitudinally and acts as the principal load-bearing member, relatively little force is generated in the direction of the X and Y axes. With segmental spinal instrumentation, the applied force is exerted by the tension in the laminar wires. Because of their orientation, these wires distribute the force primarily in the direction of the X and Y axes, with relatively little force applied in the Z direction. Therefore, the basic theoretical difference between the two methods is that the major components of applied force are perpendicular, with distraction techniques most effective in the Z direction and segmental techniques most effective in the X and Y directions.

Recognizing that the applied corrective forces of the Harrington distraction method and the Luque method are perpendicular, their respective moment arms in

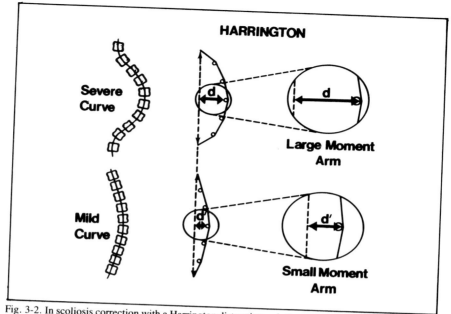

Fig. 3-2. In scoliosis correction with a Harrington distraction rod, the moment arm is *perpendicular* to the longitudinal axis of the spine. As scoliosis is corrected by this method, the effective moment arm length *decreases*, making further correction less efficient. (From Wenger: Spine Vol. 7, No. 3:260-264, 1982.)

the frontal plane must be perpendicular as well. Since segmental instrumentation applies forces in approximately the same orientation at each level undergoing instrumentation, we can simplify our discussion by comparing "resultant forces," which are the vector sum of each individual wire tension. In this way, all correction forces induced by wire attachment can be viewed as a single transverse force and a single perpendicular moment arm.

The implications of perpendicular moment arms in the frontal plane can be determined by observing the change in the basic geometry of a scoliotic curve as it is corrected. The perpendicular distance from the midline to any specific point on the curve decreases with a decrease in the measured Cobb angle. The effective moment arm present in the Harrington method is parallel to this distance; thus, the moment arm length decreases with curve correction (Fig. 3-2).

Since the bending moment required to maintain curve correction is the product of the effective moment arm and the force applied, decreasing the moment arm necessitates an increase in the longitudinally applied force. Therefore, theoretically, the Harrington distraction rod becomes mechanically less efficient in providing frontal plane correction as the curve is reduced.

In contrast, with progressive correction of the curve, the Luque method becomes theoretically more efficient in providing further correction because the longitudinally oriented effective moment arm increases in length as the curve is

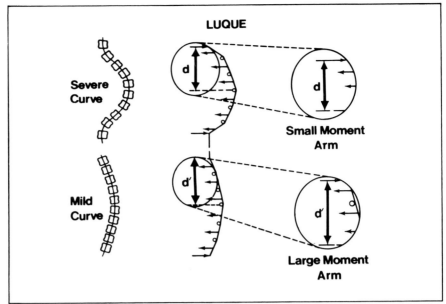

Fig. 3-3. In scoliosis correction with Luque's segmental method, the moment arm is *parallel* to the longitudinal axis of the spine. As scoliosis is corrected by this method, the effective moment arm length *increases,* making further correction more efficient. (From Wenger: Spine Vol. 7, No. 3:260-264, 1982.)

corrected (Fig. 3-3). This increases the efficiency of the force application in the frontal plane by generating a large corrective bending moment about the Y-axis without significantly increasing the force.

Because these two methods of correction are inversely related, there should be a theoretical point at which the two methods are equally effective in providing frontal plane correction. The calculated transition point at which distraction and transverse fixation supply the same bending moment when equal forces are applied (ie, equal effective moment arms) is approximately 44° of scoliosis, which compares well with the 53° calculated by White and Panjabi, who utilized a different conceptual approach.[14] This implies that for more severe curves, a Harrington distraction system would be more effective in applying the initial corrective force. However, since many scoliotic curves are reduced to less than 44°, further correction and maintenance of correction could theoretically be best achieved with segmental spinal instrumentation.

Sagittal Plane Correction

White, Panjabi, and Thomas attributed the efficiency of the Harrington distraction rod in correcting kyphosis to its ability to provide not only longitudinal distraction but also three-point bending in the sagittal plane.[15] These two force systems complement each other and, therefore, produce a large corrective bending moment about the X axis. In fact, the magnitude of the sagittal plane moment is so large that unwanted deformity (loss of thoracic kyphosis or lumbar lordosis) may be inadvertently produced in an attempt to achieve maximal frontal plane scoliosis correction with the Harrington distraction method.[8]

The standard recommendation for use of Luque's method includes contouring the readily malleable 4.8-mm ($\frac{3}{16}''$) rods to maintain sagittal contour.[2,4] Wiring the precontoured rods at every level increases the probability of maintaining near-normal thoracic kyphosis and lumbar lordosis. Such rod contouring can be performed without seriously affecting the direction of force application and therefore can be utilized without sacrificing frontal plane correction. The Harrington rod can be contoured; however, because correction is by distraction, the sagittal plane gain (maintenance of normal contour) reduces the ability to apply large forces in the frontal plane. As a result, attempts to maintain normal sagittal plane contour with the Harrington system are made at the expense of frontal plane correction. The intimate relationship between the Harrington rod's effect in the frontal and sagittal planes illustrates that correction by a single distraction rod is geometry limited. Increased distraction to achieve maximum frontal plane correction requires increasingly larger forces. As maximum correction is approached, sagittal plane enlongation increases, thereby reducing the effectiveness of correction. The end result is that any further increase in rod force provides no additional frontal plane correction. Schulz and Hirsch used computer simulation to test this hypothesis and found that for one of their model spines (NE1, 64° right thoracolumbar curve), the curve could not be corrected to less than 41°, no matter what distraction force was applied.[8] By comparison, Luque's segmental method, which utilizes transversely applied forces and sagittally contoured rods, is not geometry limited and has greater potential for achieving correction.

Rotational Correction in the Transverse Plane

The Harrington distraction rod has little, if any, mechanical effect on producing bending moments about the Z axis to correct transverse plane deformity because its longitudinal line of action does not produce the force components in the X and Y direction required for transverse plane derotation.[9] The addition of the Harrington compression system has only a mild effect on correcting rotation because its line of action is also longitudinal. Much of the apparent rib hump reduction achieved with a compression system is due to the production of thoracic lordosis, which forces the entire rib cage forward, rather than truly derotating the vertebra (and attached ribs).

Luque's method has some potential for derotation because the wire forces on the concave side contribute to the corrective bending moment. However, potential derotation depends on application of manual force to the trunk during properly sequenced wire tightening. Thus, the segmental method may be effective in maintaining a spine that has been manually derotated but does not provide specific effective derotational corrective forces in its own right.

Biomechanics of Failure

Comparison of the force that can be generated by the various methods of instrumentation is of little value without an analysis of the metal-bone interface, because the actual correction achieved depends on how effectively the applied corrective forces are transferred to the spinal column. In this context, failure is defined as fracture at the metal-bone interface, leading to loss of correction. The stress that causes this failure can be attributed to two factors: (1) the amount of force applied to the fixation site and (2) the effective area over which this force is distributed.

Fixation Sites and Their Effect

Basic structural mechanics suggests that increasing the number of supports in a structure reduces the load that each support must carry independently. Thus, in correcting scoliosis, increasing the number of fixation points not only distributes the load more evenly, but also provides increased stability of the entire instrumentation-spine complex. Therefore, Luque's method, with fixation at every level, should provide excellent acute stability and maintenance of correction, in contrast to the Harrington technique, which has only two heavily loaded fixation points.

The type of metal-bone attachment is also important because the geometry of the fixation determines the effective surface area over which the load is applied. When a standard Harrington hook (#1253) is properly inserted under the lamina, the relative surface area is considerably larger than that of the 18-gauge (1.22 mm diameter) stainless steel wires commonly used in Luque's method. However, the cumulative surface area of two wires passed under every lamina within the curve (average of ten segments) is larger than the surface area of a single Harrington hook. (The comparison is made to a single hook because the Harrington rod applies a colinear force at both hook sites; thus, each hook individually must carry the entire distractive force.) Since stress is defined as force per unit area, a constant corrective force would induce a higher stress at the hook site in the Harrington method than at any wire in the Luque system, assuming the same force were required in each method to maintain correction.

We previously mentioned that owing to the geometry-limited nature of the Harrington system, a larger force is required to maintain correction as a scoliotic curve is corrected than in the Luque method. This further increases the chance that a force limit will be reached by the Harrington method, because at some point the lamina will no longer sustain the applied load. The existence of this force limit has been generally accepted by other authors.[8,11,14]

Laboratory Testing

After developing theoretical concepts concerning segmental spinal instrumentation, we developed a laboratory model to test our hypothesis. We elected to study acute failure with an in vitro laboratory model to compare the acute stability provided by four types of scoliosis instrumentation, beginning with simple Harrington instrumentation and progressing to complex segmental instrumentation (Luque).

After reviewing previous studies by Sue-A-Quan and consulting with veterinary anatomists regarding spinal contour and facet orientation, the Holstein calf spine was selected as an in vitro model.[10] An animal model was used because fresh human spines are difficult to obtain and, when available, vary greatly in bony density because of osteoporosis, thus introducing a significant variable. In contrast, spines from one-month-old Holstein calves of a similar size provide a consistent bone density, essential for comparing acute failure of the spine instrumentation complex.

The scoliosis simulator was developed and revised based on the simulator used by Sue-A-Quan, Garside and Simmons in Toronto.[10] The spines in our study were mounted at both ends with a polyurethane foam, which provided rigid mounting of the pelvis and upper thoracic spine. A geared crank system allowed incremental shortening of the instrumentation-spine complex in the axial direction, thus progressively loading the instrumented spine. A 1000-pound load cell (force transducer) attached to a microprocessor provided serial digital readout of pounds of force of the instrumentation complex from initial load to failure.

The mounted spines were loaded to produce 30° of scoliosis in the anteroposterior (transverse) plane. Corrective instrumentation was then applied from the fourth thoracic to the third lumbar vertebra, with the applied load further adjusted so that at initiation of testing, each spine had a consistent degree of scoliosis (20°) and load (approximately 15 pounds). The instrumentation-spine complex was then axially loaded to failure of the system.

In addition, the simulator was adapted to evaluate failure in forward bending by vertically mounting the spines with the pelvis firmly fixed and the proximal spinal column free. By use of an adapter and torque wrench, a standardized forward bend was applied to the instrumented spines with degrees of bend and inch-pounds of torque at failure recorded.

A total of 54 calf spines underwent instrumentation and were tested. The systems tested included (Fig. 3-4):

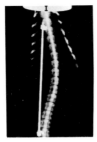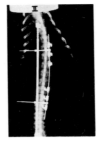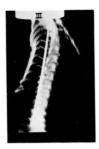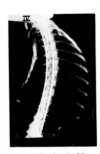

Fig. 3-4. Radiographs of calf spines undergoing instrumentation by four different methods: I. Harrington distraction; II. Harrington distraction plus compression plus transverse approximators; III. Harrington distraction plus segmental laminar wires; IV. Luque "L" rods plus segmental laminar wires. (From Wenger: Spine Vol. 7, No. 3:265-269, 1982.)

I.   Simple Harrington distraction instrumentation;

II.   Harrington distraction plus compression instrumentation connected by two transverse approximators;

III.   Single Harrington distraction rod with #1253 hooks plus 1.22-mm (18 gauge) laminar wire fixation; and

IV.   Luque segmental fixation with 4.8-mm (³⁄₁₆″) double-L rods plus 1.22-mm (18 gauge) laminar wires.

Tests in Longitudinal Compressive Loading

Sixteen spines were tested, with four in each group. The mean load to failure with each system tested is reported in Figure 3-5. Failure occurred with the lowest load (93 pounds) with simple Harrington distraction instrumentation. The applied longitudinal forces produced spinal deformity (kyphosis), which transferred a transverse load onto the midsection of the rod. This transverse force produced a three-point bending moment, which resulted in laminar fracture at either the upper (thoracic) or lower hook site (Fig. 3-6). Failure was always at the metal-bone interface.

Systems II (distraction plus compression plus transverse approximators) and III (Harrington distraction plus laminar wires) both failed at a load approximately double that used to produce failure in the Harrington distraction rod alone. These systems loaded more rapidly because the spine deformed very little with loading (less kyphosis) owing to multiple fixation points.

System IV (Luque rods plus laminar wires) failed in compression at a mean of 134 pounds; however, the mode of failure was always bending of the double rod-spine complex. In no case was there failure at the instrumentation-bone interface. Since two Luque 4.8-mm (³⁄₁₆″) rods withstand less longitudinal loading than does

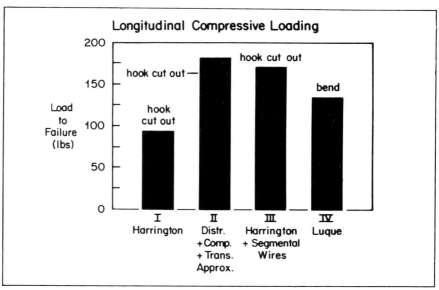

Fig. 3-5. Results of tests in compressive loading. The addition of various types of transverse fixation improved the ability of the spine-instrumentation complex to withstand acute loading. The mode of failure is listed at the top of each column. (From Wenger: Spine Vol. 7, No. 3:265-269, 1982.)

a single 6.3-mm (¼″) Harrington rod, bending began at 120 pounds and loaded only to 134 pounds (elastic limit). Further load produced only greater deformity, but no increase in measured load.

Tests in Forward Bending

The degree of forward bend and the inch-pounds of torque until failure were tested in 21 spines. The results in inch-pounds of torque at failure are reported in Figure 3-7.

Thirteen spines underwent System I instrumentation and were tested. Failure occurred at a mean of 54° of flexion, with either fracture of the thoracic facet or the hook sliding out of the facet of the uppermost instrumented vertebra. In one test, fracture-dislocation at the upper hook site occurred. Kyphotic deformity within the instrumented segment contributed to failure. The mean torque at failure was 44 inch-pounds.

Four tests were performed on spines with system II instrumentation. Spines tested in this mode failed at the upper end with a mean 39° bend and 50 inch-pounds of torque. Failure occurred with fracture-dislocation at the upper end in half the tests and with facet fracture in the remaining tests.

Systems III and IV performed identically in the four tests. Failure occurred at a mean of 45° of bend with a mean of 62.5 inch-pounds of torque; thus, there was

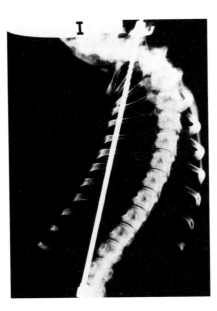

Fig. 3-6. Radiograph demonstrating facet fracture with loss of upper hook fixation seen when the Harrington distraction rod alone (System I) was applied and tested in longitudinal compressive loading. (From Wenger: Spine Vol. 7, No. 3:265-269, 1982.)

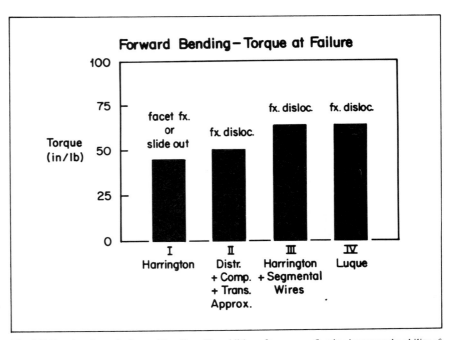

Fig. 3-7. Results of tests in forward bending. The addition of transverse fixation improves the ability of the spine-instrumentation complex to withstand an applied force. The mode of failure is noted at the top of each column. (From Wenger: Spine Vol. 7, No. 3:265-269, 1982.)

an improvement in performance as compared with Harrington distraction alone. Failure was by fracture-dislocation at the upper end in each case.

Interpretation of In Vitro Study

This in vitro simulation has led us to several conclusions regarding scoliosis correction and maintenance by the Harrington distraction rod versus Luque's segmental fixation method. First, the kyphosis that develops when a Harrington rod-spine complex is longitudinally loaded or flexed (forward bending) is minimized by the addition of transverse fixation. The added fixation points prevent the development of kyphosis with longitudinal loading, thus avoiding a transverse force on the midsection of the rod, which results in a three-point bending force system. This bending moment is a probable important cause of hook cutout with Harrington distraction instrumentation alone.

In this study, failure with the Harrington method was always accompanied by fracture at the hook-bone interface, with a resulting loss of correction within the instrumented segment. In contrast, the Luque method of segmental fixation failed outside the instrumented segment, thus maintaining correction.

The primary conclusions to be drawn from this testing are that the addition of multiple fixation sites, by whatever means, increases the ability of an instrumentation method to maintain correction, and that transversely applied forces create corrective bending in a more efficient manner than those produced by longitudinal distraction.[12]

Summary

Analysis of the biomechanics of scoliosis *correction* in the frontal plane suggests that owing to the orientation of the moment arm, the Harrington method would be theoretically more effective in correcting large curves, while the Luque method would most effectively correct mild curves.

In the sagittal plane, distraction with a straight Harrington rod may result in the loss of normal thoracic kyphosis and lumbar lordosis. Contouring a distraction rod may help in maintaining normal sagittal plane curvature, but it significantly decreases the amount of distractive force that the rod can produce, thereby reducing the ability of the system to produce frontal plane correction. In contrast, with the Luque method, properly contoured rods maintain normal sagittal plane curvature yet remain effective in providing frontal plane correction.

The relative ease with which longitudinal compressive loading produced bending of the two 4.8-mm ($^3/_{16}$″) L rods attached to the spine in the Luque method was surprising. This bending occurred more readily (134 pounds) than did that of the spines that were segmentally wired to the 6.3-mm (¼″) Harrington rod (System III). Since bending of the double-rod complex has not occurred in scoliosis patients surgically corrected with the Luque method, the bending is not interpreted as undesirable. More rigid 6.3-mm (¼″) Luque rods (which are available for the treatment of fracture-dislocation) would be more resistant to bending with longitudinal loading but could provide excessively rigid internal fixation, thus preventing the development of a strong fusion mass (to our knowledge, the concept of stress shielding in spinal instrumentation has not been addressed).

Rotational correction in the transverse plane cannot be provided by the longitudinally applied forces of the Harrington system. Although theoretically the Luque method could provide rotational correction, the position of the wire attachment and the deformity of the posterior elements limit effective derotation.

A study of the biomechanics of *failure* indicates that Luque's method, with multiple fixation points and lower stress at the attachments, provides greater stability than the Harrington system, therefore allowing a greater corrective moment to be applied.

Laboratory testing has demonstrated that added fixation greatly improves the ability to withstand acutely applied forces. One reason for this improvement is that the added fixation points prevent the development of deformity within the instrumented segment. This deformity is one factor that initiates hook cutout when longitudinal compressive, rotational, or bending loads are applied.

Despite these specific theoretical advantages in providing correction, the greatest advantage of segmental instrumentation seems to be maintaining correction rather than providing it. This is best explained by evaluating the limiting factor of both instrumentation methods. The Harrington system is geometry limited in the amount of bending moment that can be produced, which necessitates an asymptomatic increase in force to maintain maximum correction. This force increase is ultimately force-limited by the mechanical strength of the vertebral elements to which the rod is attached. The Luque method is not geometry limited and, in fact, benefits structurally from further curve reduction. Furthermore, once correction is achieved by this method, the smaller the residual curve, the lower the stress at each fixation point; therefore, correction is more easily maintained. For this method, the point at which correction should be maintained must be determined from neurologic considerations rather than from a structural standpoint.

Editor's Commentary

Dr. Wenger's work has become a classic. Nevertheless, several points have remained unclear because of lack of extensive laboratory experimentation. For

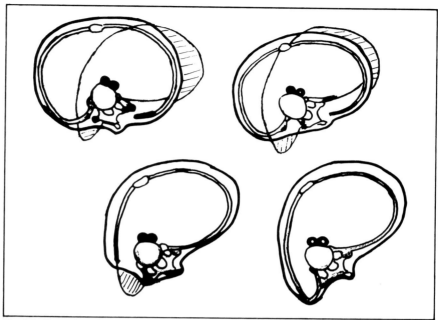

Fig. 3-8. Correction of apical rotation must include elimination of not only bony deformities, eg, in the chest (segmental rings around vertebrae, ribs, and sternum) but also soft tisse contractures, such as annular disk ligaments and other paravertebral structures.

Bottom right, axial view of thoracic ring deformity.

Bottom left, correction of the deformed thoracic ring by rib resection on the convex side of the deformity.

Upper right, correction of thoracic ring by osteotomy of concave rib and convex transverse process; partial "derotation" of the rib cage. Notice no change in the rotational deformity of the vertebra, only transposition of the midline.

Upper left, complete correction of thoracic ring by complete release of soft tissues above and below that segmental thoracic ring. Osteotomies of the concave side of the ring (concave rib) and of the convex side of the ring (convex transverse process) permit the rib on that side to rotate as the corresponding vertebra is derotated and transposed to the midline.

example, the statement "due to the orientation of the moment arm, the Harrington method would be theoretically more effective in correcting large curves, while the Luque method would be most effective in correcting mild curves" is a fallacy, since in this study Wenger states "with SSI, the applied force is exerted by the tension in the laminar wires." The forces of correction in SSI include not only transverse traction but also (and very importantly) pressure over the apex and lateral bend, which is not even mentioned, created as the flexible ends are brought into alignment from the pressure of the concave bar and transverse traction of the convex bar.[18] Of course, this can only be true if both bars are united to form a complete force.[18] Therefore, the corrective forces of SSI have not really been tested, and the original statement cannot be valid. Only one of four corrective forces has been presumed in SSI, and that is transverse traction. On the other hand, this merely represents the complexity of the system. The only way to analyze it is

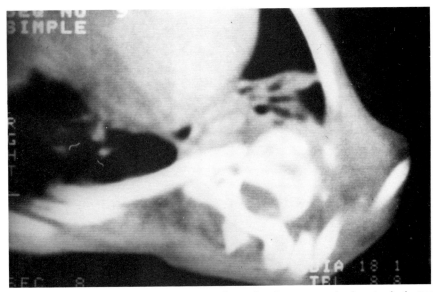

Fig. 3-9. CAT scan projection of an apical scoliotic vertebra demonstrates clearly not only the true degree of rotation (32°) and vertebral deformity but also the immense deformity of the thoracic cage. In the convex side, no room is left for any anatomic structures, because the rib deformity is extreme. On the concave side, the pathologic insertion of the rib is a bony strut that impedes any type of physiologic correction of the deformity.

by looking at the corrective forces individually. These are then combined in a total analysis of the entire system before a definitive statement is made.

It is most important to assert that distraction leads to correction in one single plane. To maintain normal sagittal curves or even dream of apical derotation is a fantasy. These corrections, of course, depend on segmental correctability, and this in turn depends on segmental bony pathology and soft tissue contractures.

As for apical rotation, it has been my personal clinical experience that only by doing diskectomies and parting the segmental ring in two places (concave rib and convex transverse process) can actual derotation take place (Fig. 3-8).

It is very nice to assume theoretically that pressure from the convex bar at the apex and posterolateral traction in that same segment, exerted by the concave bar and corresponding sublaminar wires, will produce a torque moment that will produce derotation. In practice, this is not true for several reasons. (1) There is an interfacet bony black posterior. (2) There is a wedged deformed vertebral body in front. (3) There is an ankylosed annular ligament in both the cephalic and the caudal disk. (4) There is a "ring" deformity in the transverse plane. (5) There is intersegmental deformity, which includes both anterior and posterior longitudinal ligaments plus all the paravertebral musculature and ligamentous interconnections (Fig. 3-9).

It is also important to note that in the "state of the art," the Cobb angle means very little, since it measures only the end vertebral plates, where the deformity is minimal. Some very important pathologic factors, such as posterior element deformity, apical vertebra deformity, apical rotation, sagittal deformity, flexibility of the soft tissue deformity, and overall three-dimensional balance of a curve have been ignored.

I would like to point out that these studies have been done with double-L 3/16-inch rods with No. 18 gauge wire; nothing has been done with 1/4-inch rods or other configurations now more commonly in use, like C or rectangle rods or U or rhomboid antirotational rods. Different strengths of wire and wire twisting, eg, double wires with hooks and wire twist over bars, have only started to appear in recent studies.

No research has been done concerning the use of SSI as a temporary structural replacement of spinal bony structure. Its role as a supportive structure in a collapsing spine and its relation to metal rigidity and bony plasticity must also be studied. Other study topics include the effect of total rigidity on partial flexibility, and metallic failure during continuous stress and movement, as in a growing child without an arthrodesis or external support.

More than any other chapter in this book, this one fully explains "SSI, The State of The Art."

References

1. Belytschko TB, Anriacchi TP, Schultz AB, Galante JO: Analog studies of forces in the human spine: Computational techniques. J Biomech 6:361-371, 1973.

2. Ferguson RL, Allen BL: Segmental spinal instrumentation for routine scoliotic curve. Contemp Ortho 2:450-454, 1980.

3. Gross C, Graham J, Neuwirth M, Pugh J: Scoliosis and growth, an analysis of the literature. Clin Ortho 175:243-250, 1983.

4. Luque ER, Cardosa A: Segmental Correction of Scoliosis with Rigid Internal Fixation. Presented at the annual meeting of the Scoliosis Research Society, Ottawa, Ontario, Canada, September 6, 1976.

5. Panjabi MM: Three-dimensional mathematical model of the human spine structure. J Biomech 6:671-680, 1973.

6. Resina J, Alves AF: A technique of correction and internal fixation for scoliosis. J Bone Jt Surg 59B:159-165, 1977.

7. Schultz AB, Hirsch C: Mechanical analysis of Harrington rod correction of idiopathic scoliosis. J Bone Jt Surg 55A:983-992, 1973.

8. Schultz AB, Hirsch C: Mechanical analysis of techniques for improved correction of idiopathic scoliosis. Clin Ortho 100:66-73, 1974.

9. Schultz AB: A biomechanical view of scoliosis. Spine 1:162-271, 1976.

10. Sue-A-Quan EA: Anterior Instrumentation of Spine. Thesis for Master of Surgery, University of Toronto, Toronto, Ontario, Canada, August, 1970.

11. Waugh RT: Intravital measurements during instrumental correction of idiopathic scoliosis. Acta Ortho Scand (Suppl) 93:1-87, 1966.

12. Wenger DR, Carollo JJ, Wilkerson JA: Biomechanics of scoliosis correction by segmental spinal instrumentation. Spine 7:260-264, 1982.

13. Wenger DR, Carollo JJ, Wilkerson JA, Wauters K, Herring JA: Laboratory testing of segmental spinal instrumentation versus traditional Harrington instrumentation for scoliosis treatment. Spine 7:265-269, 1982.

14. White AA, Panjabi MM: The clinical biomechanics of scoliosis. Clin Ortho 118:100-112, 1976.

15. White AA, Panjabi MM, Thomas CL: The clinical biomechanics of kyphotic deformities. Clin Ortho 128:8-17, 1977.

16. White AA, Panjabi MM: Clinical biomechanics of the spine. Philadelphia, JB Lippincott, 1978, pp 91-114.

17. Luque ER: Metodos para medir escoliosis. Revista Mexicana de Radiologia. No. 4. Julio-Agosto, 1968.

18. Luque ER: Segmental Correction and Fixation of the Spine. Exhibit, American Academy of Orthopaedic Surgeons, Dallas, Texas, 1978.

Indications, Patient Selection, and Evaluation in Pediatric Orthopedics

4

Principles

CERTAIN BASIC PRINCIPLES ARE EMPHASIZED in this chapter. The first is that the best instrumentation and the finest surgical technique must be subordinate to sound clinical judgment based on a carefully obtained history and physical examination. Also we stress that the art of decision-making is far harder to teach than is surgical technique.

Another area emphasized is comprehensive preoperative planning. Such planning must include consideration of the patient's overall medical and neurologic status. Management of pulmonary problems and seizure disorders must begin preoperatively. The anesthesia team should be included in planning surgery for any complicated situation so that hypotensive anesthesia, spinal cord monitoring, and other special techniques may be considered.

In planning surgical correction, the surgeon must assess the spine relative to

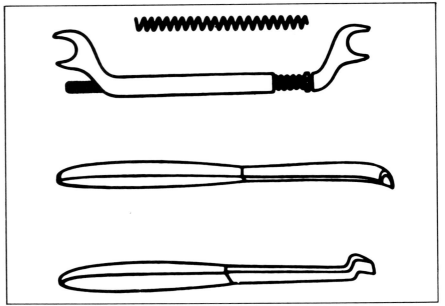

Fig. 4-1. A distraction device first described by Gruca of Poland in 1958.

its three-dimensional contour. The surgeon must compile his data (physical examination, plane radiographs, CT scans, and so forth) to evaluate the deformity based on three components, ie, the sagittal curves, the postural curves, and the pelvic obliquity. He must understand the disease entity he is treating and the spinal changes likely to be present. There is tremendous variability among the disorders lumped together as neurogenic scoliosis, and successful management involves understanding those differences. The spine of a severely athetoid, muscular teenager bears little resemblance to the fragile spine of the youngster with spinal muscular atrophy.

A number of anatomic principles also need emphasis. The biomechanical properties of the vertebrae have been studied by Harrington, Wenger, and Luque.[3,5,6] In all these studies, the strongest posterior structure has been found to be the neural arch. To obtain maximum stability, instrumentation must be firmly attached to the lamina-pedicle complex. Attachment of instrumentation to the spinous processes affords only a fraction of the strength of fixation available with fixation to the neural arch. This becomes especially important in dealing with the osteopenic spine.

Another important principle is that instrumentation does not correct a spinal deformity beyond its degree of passive flexibility. Thus, the flexibility of a curve demonstrated on passive bending radiographs is indicative of the maximal correction that can be obtained by internal fixation alone. In order to correct a fixed deformity, release of contracted structures on the concavity of the deformity and shortening of structures on the convexity of the deformity will be necessary.

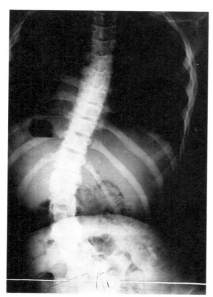

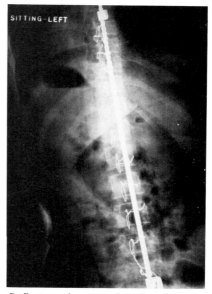

Fig. 4-2. A 17-year-old boy with posttraumatic paraplegia.

A, Preoperative anteroposterior radiograph showing a scoliosis of 42 degrees.

B, Postoperative correction of scoliosis to 0 degrees with Harrington instrumentation and laminar wiring.

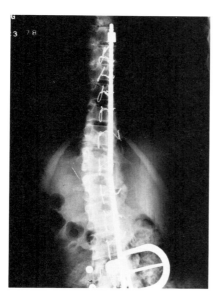

C, Radiograph 25 months postoperatively showing a fracture of the rod associated with pseudarthrosis.

In addition to having an awareness of basic principles, the surgeon must be expert in the use of a variety of techniques in order to use the system correctly. He must be able to contour rods to produce appropriate correction and maintain postural curves. He must be able to obtain firm pelvic fixation when necessary. He must also be familiar with techniques applicable to the myelodysplastic spine so that adequate fixation to the pedicles can be accomplished. Finally, he must know when to innovate. In dealing with highly complex and variable deformities, the need to improvise will be inevitable. This instrumentation system owes much of its usefulness to the many changes that began as original maneuvers when known techniques were inadequate.

Patient Evaluation

History

The history of illness has long been the cornerstone of clinical medicine. Physicians and surgeons are constantly tempted by the sparkling marvels of medical science to omit or abbreviate this most important segment of patient care. Yet, in the long run, more false steps are avoided and more traps eluded by attention to this one simple task than to any other.

Children are both excellent and terrible historians; the chosen view often reflects the skill of the examiner. A child answers "no" when asked if he has pain. The same child, when asked to point to where it hurts, will often do so willingly. A child may state that his back never hurts. On the other hand, if asked, he will admit that it "gets tired" at the end of the day and he has to lie down. It is taught that stocking anesthesia is a hysterical symptom. Frequently, however, the patient with severe spondylolistheses will voice just such a complaint. We are taught that scoliosis does not hurt and thus ignore the fact that half our patients say that their back aches at the apex of the curve. Attention to the pattern of pain may allow us to anticipate the presence of spinal tumor, spondylolisthesis, herniated disk, or osteoid osteoma.

An especially important segment of the history is the neurologic evaluation. It is wise to begin with the history of cortical, cerebellar, cranial nerve, motor, and sensory systems before focusing on the obvious complaint of a curved spine. The subtle sensory and motor changes of syringomyelia may be completely missed unless sought out. The fact that one foot requires a smaller shoe than the other may be the only finding noticed by the patient with a diastematomyelia. A history of bowel and bladder function is essential in ruling out subtle neurologic deficits.

An area most often neglected by orthopedic surgeons is the review of systems. We should not be amazed that the parent forgot to tell us about a bleeding episode in the dentist's office—it's our job to ask. One should keep a mental (or actual) checklist which includes malignant hyperthermia, allergies, hemorrhage, urinary

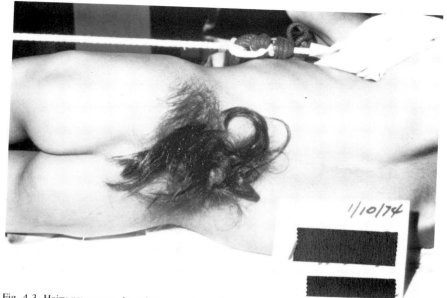

Fig. 4-3. Hairy nevus over the spine in a patient with diastematomyelia.

dysfunction, and drug use, to name a few. Likewise, the family history may provide valuable diagnostic clues. The severity of disease in another affected family member may be one's best prognostic indicator in conditions such as Charcot-Marie-Tooth syndrome, osteogenesis imperfecta, or neurofibromatosis.

Physical Examination

The general examination is often the most important of the entire physical examination. From this segment of the examination, we ascertain the patient's nutritional status, his cooperativeness, his mood, and his habitus. Any signs of dwarfism should alert the examiner to the possibility of cervical anomalies such as hypoplasia of the odontoid in truncal dwarfing conditions such as spondyloepiphyseal dysplasia. With the extremity dwarfing of achondroplasia, we become aware of the problems associated with a narrowed, sometimes kyphotic spinal canal.

The examination of the skin should also be carefully performed. Certain rashes such as pediculosis may seriously confound postoperative management. The presence of impetigo anywhere on the skin significantly increases the risk of a wound infection. Cafe au lait spots are often the clue to neurofibromatosis. Any skin lesion, from a hemangioma to a hairy nevus, when located over the spine is an indicator of possible spinal dysraphism (Fig. 4-3).

In the examination of the head, eyes, ears, nose, and throat, certain special considerations should be noted. The presence of a subcutaneous cerebrospinal fluid shunt should be noted, and the physician should ascertain if it is functional. It also reminds the physician of the necessity for prophylactic antibiotic coverage using an agent that penetrates the cerebrospinal fluid. An unusual frontal prominence of the skull may be the indicator of cleidocranial dysostosis. A bluish tint to the sclerae suggests osteogenesis imperfecta, some cases of which are unrecognized because of their mild nature. The nose and throat are examined for evidence of upper respiratory infection. In the diastrophic dwarf, the muscles that elevate the palate are deficient, and this is often associated with middle ear infection. In the arthrogrypotic, there may be pharyngeal muscle dysfunction, which may cause postoperative aspiration and death.

The physical examination of the thorax can often be as helpful as pulmonary function tests. The ability to cough, take a deep breath, blow out a match, and hold the breath should be tested. The anteroposterior diameter of the chest correlates well with vital capacity. In the severely handicapped, the clearance of respiratory secretions should be noted.

The cardiac and abdominal examinations are necessary to rule out other unsuspected abnormalities. Weak abdominal musculature associated with neurologic disease may also suggest future respiratory and renal difficulties.

A standard neurologic examination is an essential part of the work-up of the patient. A useful series of tests of motor function consists of having the patient heel walk, toe walk, hop on one foot, and get up from the floor. If the patient can do all these without difficulty, there is little likelihood of a significant lower extremity motor weakness. If the patient then can walk a straight line heel to toe, stand still with his eyes closed, and do the finger to nose test, he is unlikely to have a disorder of the cerebellum or posterior columns. The spine surgeon should be especially watchful for the atrophic calf and the short or cavus foot of spinal dysraphism. An examination cannot be complete if the patient does not remove his shoes and socks!

The surgeon now is free to approach the spinal examination, and he does so with certain things in mind. He not only will assess the existing deformity, but will also constantly ask himself how he is to improve upon it. Especially important is the overall alignment. The examination begins with observation of the patient standing unclothed. Is the head centered over the pelvis? Are the shoulders level? Are the leg lengths equal? Is there evidence of pelvic obliquity? The same points should be noted as the patient walks. With forward bending, the curve rotation and flexibility are noted. The postural curves are also noted and are evaluated for flexibility. It is especially important not only to note the absence of thoracic kyphosis but also to determine if any kyphosis returns when the patient bends forward. The flexibility of minor curves should also be noted.

The spinal examination is incomplete without an examination of the hips. Abduction and adduction contractures are often unrecognized initiators and perpetuators of spinal deformity. The best spine surgery in the world cannot correct pelvic obliquity if it is fixed below the pelvis. Many apparently neurogenic curves will regress when a subluxated hip is corrected.

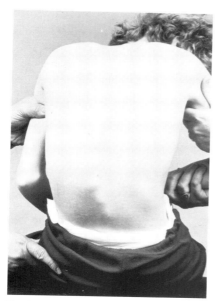

Fig. 4-4. A patient with severe athetoid cerebral palsy.

A, Sitting posture showing slumping kyphosis.

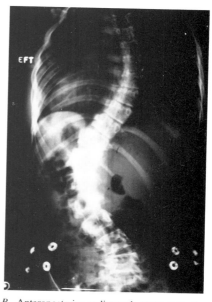

B, Anteroposterior radiograph preoperatively showing a 70 degree curve.

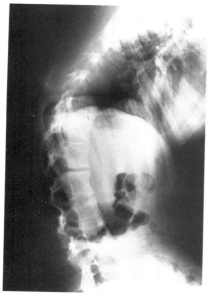

C, Preoperative lateral radiograph showing a slumping kyphosis of 51 degrees.

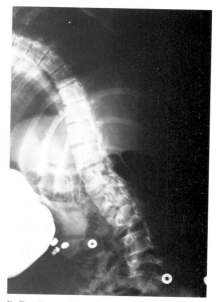

D, Bending radiograph with curve correction to 24 degrees.

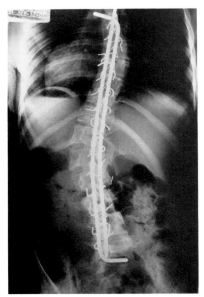 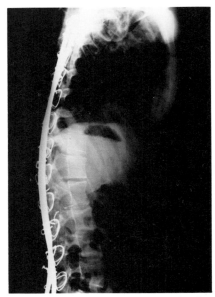

E, Postoperative anteroposterior radiograph with the curve corrected to 48 degrees.

F, Postoperative lateral radiographs showing correction of the kyphotic curve to 20 degrees.

Laboratory Examination

A general baseline evaluation should include a complete blood count, urinalysis, and clotting factor screening. Pulmonary function tests, electrocardiograms, and chest radiographs are often indicated. Any tests necessary to clarify or establish a diagnosis should be performed preoperatively.

Radiographic Examination

Plain anteroposterior and lateral radiographs should be taken with the patient upright. The head and pelvis should be included in order to evaluate truncal alignment. We obtain bending films by having the patient lie supine while forceful correction of the curve is done by another person (Fig. 4-4). To evaluate the flexibility of kyphotic curves, the patient lies supine on a firm bolster, and a lateral radiograph is taken. To evaluate the flexibility of thoracic hypokyphosis, the patient lies prone on a bolster placed against the sternum, while a lateral radiograph is taken (Fig. 4-5). With some spinal deformities, such as congenital scoliosis, tomography is helpful in defining vertebral anatomy. With other deformities, computerized axial tomography (CAT) may better define the vertebral structure. When spinal dysraphism is a possibility, as in congenital scoliosis, myelography is necessary prior to surgical correction. Myelography is also indicated when unexplained neurologic findings are present and when dural ectasia is a possibility, as in neurofibromatosis. An evaluation of ventricular size by CT scan is necessary if the status of a shunt is in question.

Preoperative Planning

By far the most important part of preoperative planning is the setting of the goals of treatment. The surgeon must always ask himself what it is that the patient needs. Another way of stating this is to ask what the risk-benefit ratio for this particular set of circumstances is. Frequently, we make the surgical decision without really taking stock of these goals and perform "triumphs of technology over reason." For sake of discussion, possible goals have been divided into three categories.

1. First, our goal may be to achieve maximum correction and stabilization. An example would be a patient with paraplegia, scoliosis, and pelvic obliquity. Total correction of the pelvic obliquity is essential to prevent future problems with decubitus ulceration. In this situation, the risks of extreme correction are small compared with the risks of leaving the deformity undercorrected.

2. Often, our goal may be limited to obtaining enough correction to level the pelvis and stabilize the curve. An example is the patient with major pulmonary compromise, such as an older patient with Duchenne's dystrophy. While maximum correction would require an anterior approach, acceptable correction may be achieved by a posterior approach alone. When the patient has intact sensation, the correction of pelvic obliquity is desirable but not as essential as in the patient with insensitive skin and predilection for pressure sores. Many times, the risks to neurologic function outweigh the need for maximum correction, as in the patient with a tethered spinal cord.

3. Another compromise goal may be to seek to stabilize a curve against further progression and achieve little if any correction. This may be the case in a severely retarded patient, one with major congenital anomalies, or one with severe osteopenia. In osteogenesis imperfecta, early instrumentation and fusion when the curve is mild may not require much correction. Fusion at this stage may be a conservative thing to do. On the other hand, fusion at a later date with a severe curve and very osteopenic bone may offer the surgeon no options for obtaining much improvement.

In planning treatment, it is a good habit first to plan the medical aspects. Planning at this stage includes pulmonary support, seizure control, blood replacement, and postoperative events. It is especially important to evaluate the likelihood of the patient's cooperating with postoperative immobilization or activity limitations.

The orthopedic (straight child) planning can best be done by considering three components of the deformity. First, the evaluation focuses on the major and minor sagittal curves. How much correction is necessary? How flexible are the curves? If the necessary correction exceeds the forced bending radiographs, will better

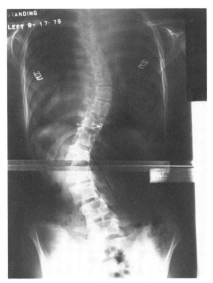

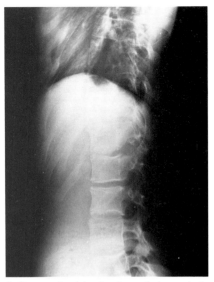

Fig. 4-5. A patient with idiopathic scoliosis and thoracic lordosis.

A, Preoperative anteroposterior radiographs showing a 46 degree scoliosis.

B, Preoperative lateral radiograph demonstrating a thoracic lordosis of 13 degrees.

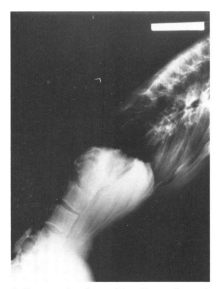

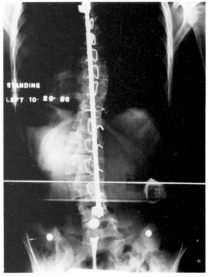

C, Preoperative forward bending radiograph showing a reduction of the thoracic lordosis to 0 degrees.

D, Postoperative anteroposterior radiograph showing the scoliosis reduced to 34 degrees with Harrington instrumentation and laminar wiring.

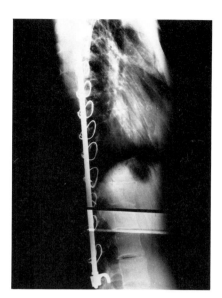

E, Postoperative lateral radiograph showing reduction of the thoracic lordosis to 0 degrees.

correction be achieved by combining an anterior procedure with a posterior one? Anterior diskectomies usually add considerable correction in the lumbar spine and moderate to minimal correction in the thoracic spine. Dwyer instrumentation adds considerably to lumbar curve correction (Fig. 4-6).

The second component of planning is that of postural curve correction or maintenance (Fig. 4-4). Ideally, the patient will have a normal degree of thoracic kyphosis and lumbar lordosis when the spine undergoes instrumentation. When the postural curves are acceptable to start, the plan should be to contour the instrumentation to maintain existing curves. One must remember that distraction posteriorly flattens lordosis. On the other hand, compression instrumentation posteriorly flattens kyphosis, while Dwyer instrumentation flattens lordosis or produces kyphosis.

When a pathologic postural curve exists, the plan should include an evaluation of that curve's flexibility. It is wishful thinking to imagine that bent rods will correct an inflexible, long-standing thoracic hypokyphosis. If thoracic hypokyphosis does not improve with forward bending, only an anterior diskectomy will allow significant correction, and that correction will depend on the remaining width of the disks.

The most difficult postural curve with which to deal is pathologic kyphosis. In our experience, the correction of kyphosis carries a significant risk of neurologic impairment. Also, kyphosis produces the greatest stresses on both the instrumentation and the neural arch. Anterior diskectomy and fusion are usually indicated for any kyphosis that will not correct to less than 50°. In correcting kyphotic curves, compression of the spinal cord and the anterior spinal artery may occur as the spine is straightened. The reason for this is that when the cord is elongated, it is also

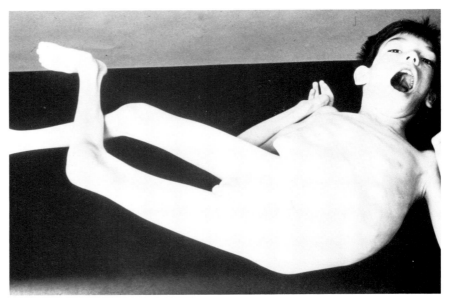

Fig. 4-6. B.B., a 16-year-old patient with severe athetoid cerebral palsy. The inability to sit was a major obstacle to his care and education.

A, Preoperative photograph showing severe scoliosis and hip extension contractures.

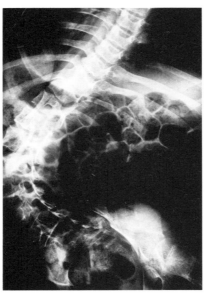

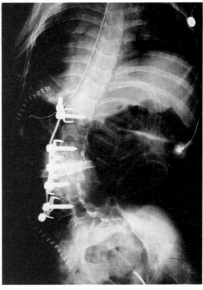

B, Preoperative anteroposterior radiograph showing a scoliosis of 107 degrees with pelvic obliquity of 75 degrees.

C, Postoperative anteroposterior radiograph following Dwyer instrumentation and fusion.

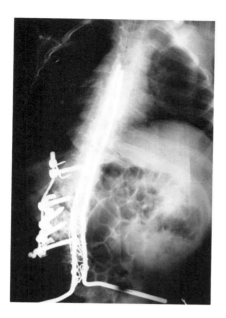

D, Anteroposterior radiograph following second-stage L-rod instrumentation and fusion to the pelvis. The scoliosis was corrected to 35 degrees and the pelvic obliquity to 10 degrees.

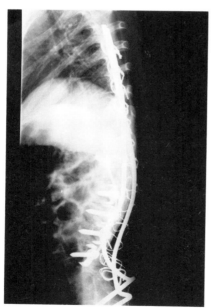

E, Postoperative views of the patient.

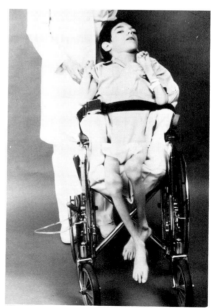

F, Now able to sit with support.

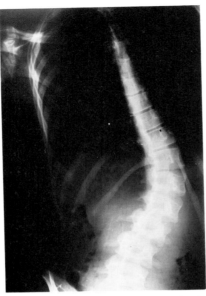

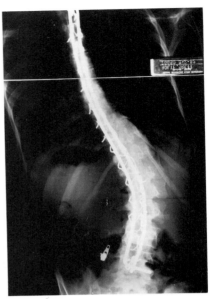

Fig. 4-7. An 18-year-old patient with athetoid cerebral palsy.

A, Preoperative anteroposterior radiograph showing a mild pelvic obliquity.

B, Anteroposterior radiograph following an L-rod instrumentation. The reduction of the fractional curve from L3 to L5 has caused increased pelvic obliquity.

pulled anteriorly against the vertebral bodies. It is the bodies that are the compressive element. When there is a neurologic deficit, decompression may be accomplished by the removal of the compressive posterior portions of the vertebral bodies.

The final stage of planning involves correction of pelvic obliquity. When there is little or no obliquity, care must be taken to avoid producing obliquity by reducing a fractional curve. In Fig. 4-7, the instrumentation resulted in increased pelvic obliquity. This occurred because the fractional curve at L3-L5 was reduced, causing the trunk to shift to the left. Proper instrument contouring would have maintained this useful curve. Frequently, reduction of the major sagittal curve adequately corrects pelvic obliquity without fusion to the pelvis. When this is accomplished, the maintenance of a mobile segment may be useful for sitting, walking, and avoiding pressure sores. When the pelvic obliquity is an integral part of the deformity (Fig. 4-6), instrumentation to the pelvis is usually necessary. The addition of an anterior fusion usually adds considerably to the correction of the obliquity. In our most recent patient series, an average of only five degrees of correction of pelvic obliquity was obtained with posterior fusion alone, compared with eighteen degrees of correction when combined anterior and posterior procedures were performed.

The next consideration is the other factors influencing treatment. First considering the osseous structures, planning is formulated relative to the strength and integrity of the spine. When there is severe osteopenia, little correction with posterior instrumentation is feasible. When the posterior elements are not present, proper instrumentation should be available to use the pedicles for fixation. When vertebral bodies are deficient, anterior strut graft placement should be considered. Congenital vertebral deformities present specific risks in approaching and performing instrumentation of the spine. Laminectomies and radiation often produce the most challenging anatomic problems.

Consideration of the soft tissues is also an important facet of planning. When there is a major midline skin and soft tissue problem, as in spina bifida, a "Y" shaped incision avoiding the abnormal area may be judicious. Soft tissue contractures should be evaluated and appropriate releases planned to achieve optimal correction. The state of the spinal cord is most important. Dr. Edward Simmons has underscored the necessity at times of even excising the dura as a contracted structure, but the author has had no experience with this approach!

Finally, there are some useful techniques in planning correction. Malleable wires placed over the bending radiographs are useful in planning rod contouring. The complex nature of rod contouring can be appreciated when the templates are also bent to match the corrected lateral radiographs in order to simulate the final three-dimensional rod contour. These template rods may be used intraoperatively to assist in contouring the L rods.

Specific Disorders

The decision to undertake major spinal surgery can never be reduced to simple consideration of degrees of curve, percentage of vital capacity, or intelligence quotient. The difficulty of this decision is magnified in the patient with major neuromuscular problems. There are no concrete answers to the questions, "When is a patient too retarded to benefit from corrective spinal surgery?" "When will a very severe curve stop progressing?" "What is the life expectancy of an individual with Duchenne's muscular dystrophy?"

The factors to be considered in the decision-making process include the likely longevity of the patient, the likely consequences of not correcting his spinal deformity, and the risks associated with such procedures. In dealing with children with severe handicaps, the opinions of the parents, therapists, and institutional caretakers are often invaluable considerations. For example, the positive feedback from parents of children with Duchenne's dystrophy has encouraged a dramatic reappraisal of surgery for this disorder.

The other difficult part of the decision-making process involves knowing when to employ and when to abandon nonoperative methods of treatment. Certainly, in the early stages, orthotic support may be useful in managing neurogenic scoliosis. Also, appropriate seating systems may even prevent the development of spinal deformity. Likewise, the importance of appropriate attention to hip stability and contractures cannot be overemphasized. On the other hand, excessive reliance upon orthotics can be detrimental. The child with osteogenesis imperfecta can be harmed by orthotics if all that happens is the production of rib deformities while a flexible curve becomes rigid.

In order to consider specific disorders relative to segmental instrumentation, the more common ones have been divided into osteopenic and nonosteopenic groups. Certain considerations in the surgical approach will apply generally to the syndromes included in each category. Many times, if these characteristics are considered in the planning stage, unfortunate outcomes may be prevented.

Osteopenic Disorders

The disorders usually characterized by moderate to extreme osteopenia include osteogenesis imperfecta, Duchenne's muscular dystrophy, spinal muscular atrophy, severe polio, high spinal cord injury, arthrogryposis, and myelodysplasia. The problems associated with Duchenne's dystrophy will serve as a prototype for discussion. The spinal deformity usually begins as a long, C-shaped, very flexible curve. In the earliest stages, it appears that the patient is only leaning excessively to one side. It is in this stage that careful attention to seating is especially important. A firm seat and a back that promotes spinal lordosis seem to be helpful. Placing the wheelchair controls in the midline may reduce the tendency of the patient to lean to one side. Orthotic devices that encase the thorax or abdomen are contraindicated because of associated pulmonary compromise.

Unfortunately, once a significant curve appears in a patient with muscular dystrophy, there is a great likelihood of further progression, often in spite of careful seating support. In managing this problem, there clearly seems to be a break-even point. One should be certain that curve progression is inevitable and should employ nonoperative support up to that point. On the other hand, each significant increase in the curve is accompanied by a corresponding decrease in flexibility and, more significantly, a decrease in vital capacity. Thus, it is reasonable to recommend surgical correction when the curve reaches 30° or 40°. At this point, the curve will be flexible, and complete correction of pelvic obliquity should be attained. Also, the patient will have sufficient pulmonary reserve to tolerate the procedure without major difficulties. Even at this early stage, careful pre- and postoperative pulmonary management is essential. In our series, we have also found that these patients may develop cardiac myopathy, so careful management of fluids is essential.

Surgical planning in this group of disorders begins with a consideration of blood loss. Osteopenic bone is usually hypermetabolic and as such has a rich blood supply. At times, in these syndromes, blood loss may be excessive. We have found the use of hypotensive anesthesia to be a major advantage in reducing bleeding. This important point should be planned in advance with anesthesia personnel, and requires intraoperative monitoring of arterial pressure.

Osteopenia presents obvious problems for instrumentation. The surgical exposure of the vertebrae has to be altered to avoid penetrating the outer cortex of the vertebrae. Sharp dissection with a forceps and knife is often safer than using a periosteal elevator. The bone consistency is similar to cardboard and, with too much pressure, will fold inward. These weak neural arches can, at times, be avulsed, when the wires are pulled beneath the laminae. Often, there is marked lumbar lordosis, making the passage of wires in the lumbar segment very difficult. Laminotomies may be necessary where the laminae overlap. In addition, contouring the rods into the lordosis may be difficult. One should avoid the tendency to try to correct the lordosis by pulling the laminae up to the rods, because the osteopenic neural arch will usually break under this force. The excessive lordosis may even be useful by transferring weightbearing forces forward to the thighs and away from the sacrum.

In these disorders, it is especially important to evaluate the bending radiographs. When the bone is weak, correction to the degree demonstrated on the bending films is often difficult to obtain; certainly, one cannot go beyond that amount. If correction beyond the bending films is desired, one must consider an anterior approach as a first stage. In Duchenne's dystrophy, this is often contraindicated because of the threat to pulmonary reserve imposed by two major operations.

Fusion to the pelvis in these disorders remains controversial. In Duchenne's dystrophy, we have usually fused to L5 and have not seen progression of pelvic obliquity. In some of the other disorders, such as high spinal cord injury, it is usually necessary to obtain sacral and pelvic stability by fusing to the pelvis. This is especially true when there is loss of sensation and when the risk of skin breakdown is great.

The choice of an upper level for instrumentation—a decision that is usually easy in the idiopathic individual—requires careful consideration in these disorders. Frequently, the upright lateral radiograph is the most useful in making this determination. The upper level of instrumentation should extend one or two levels above the top of any kyphotic curve on this lateral radiograph. In the patient with a kyphotic sitting posture, this usually means that the instrumentation must extend to the second or third thoracic vertebra. When one begins lower than this, the patient will develop subsequent kyphosis, with the apex of the curve at the upper level of instrumentation. This places the upper level under maximal stress and accounts for many of the cases of instrumentation failure.

Most of these considerations apply to the patient with spinal muscular atrophy or other severe hypotonic motor disorders. The child with osteogenesis imperfecta may present very difficult problems with osteopenic bone (Fig. 4-8). With care, even the most severely affected cases can, however, successfully undergo instrumentation and fusion. Iliac bone grafts may be so poor that they are not worth harvesting, and banked bone should be available. The patient with osteogenesis imperfecta usually has no pulmonary compromise unless the curve is quite severe, and he may be able to tolerate multiple procedures without difficulty. These children are not well managed in postoperative casts; if immobilization is necessary, synthetic casting materials are preferable to plastic jackets because of better

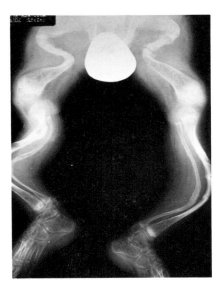

Fig. 4-8. A 6-year-old boy with severe osteogenesis imperfecta.

A, Anteroposterior radiograph of the lower extremities showing extreme bowing deformities.

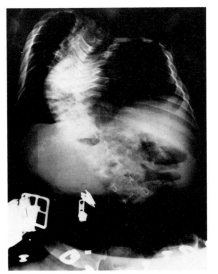

B, Anteroposterior radiograph of the spine. Scoliosis that has progressed to 77 degrees.

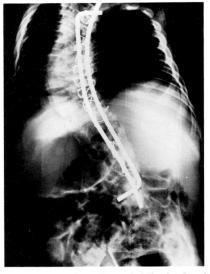

C, Anteroposterior radiograph following L-rod instrumentation and fusion, showing a scoliosis of 46 degrees.

air circulation and moisture evaporation.

The patient with myelodysplasia requires careful evaluation of urologic status as well as consideration of possibly unrecognized problems with cerebrospinal fluid dynamics. Skin condition, especially relative to previous spinal closure surgery, is very important. Frequently, a surgical approach involving a "Y" shaped incision that skirts the abnormal midline area offers the best access for instrumentation. Pelvic obliquity must be corrected to help prevent pressure sores. Anterior fusion is almost always necessary to achieve stable fusion.

The Nonosteopenic Disorders

The disorders in this category include cerebral palsy, mental retardation, congenital scoliosis, and dwarfism. The prototype for discussion will be the athetoid cerebral palsy patient (Figs. 4-4 and 4-6).

The spinal deformity in this group should again be first approached with orthotic and seating support. When instituted early, these measures may be efficacious. In the athetoid patient, external support is difficult to apply and often unsuccessful. The spinal deformity may progress quite rapidly and may early on become inflexible. There may be marked muscular hypertrophy, especially on the concavity of the curve. When the deformity is well established, muscle releases may improve curve correction.

The instrumentation of these disorders is not nearly as difficult as in the osteopenic group. The bone is not excessively vascular and is usually as strong as normal. Thus, heavy wires and rods may be used overzealously. Correction that exceeds the best bending radiograph should be avoided in order not to jeopardize spinal cord function.

These patients often tolerate multiple procedures without difficulty. When inadequate correction is produced on the bending films, consideration should be given to anterior diskectomy, Dwyer instrumentation, and fusion. As in the osteopenic diseases, there are often problems if the instrumentation does not extend to the upper thoracic levels. Instrumentation to the pelvis may be avoided if pelvic obliquity is not an integral part of the curve. When there is a major pelvic tilt, placement of rods into the ilium with fusion to the pelvis is necessary. We have not used skeletal traction in these patients in recent years, although some surgeons find this to be helpful.

In the patients in this group, very stable instrumentation is usually easily achieved. It is in these children that the avoidance of postoperative immobilization is most appreciated. The retarded child or the child with seizures, athetosis, or spasticity has major difficulties with immobilization. We have not had instrumentation failures in these patients while employing a program of nonimmobilization. We caution against vigorous activities, but these instructions are frequently impossible to enforce. Our early fears that the fixation would fail have not materialized in these patients if they have adequate bone strength.

Patients with dwarfism also are well managed with segmental systems. Awareness on the part of the anesthesia and surgical team of possible cervical instability, as well as problems in the function of the palate and pharynx, is

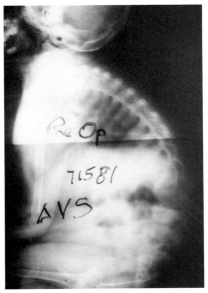 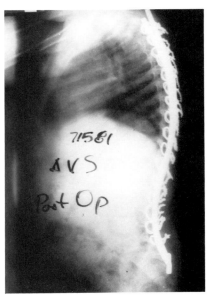

Fig. 4-9A. Male, 4 years old, with Duchenne's muscular dystrophy who cannot sit up without use of his arms (tripod sitter).

B, Same patient as Fig. 4-9A after SSI, erect with physiologic sagittal curves molded into the bars. No arthrodesis was done.

essential. Children with diastrophic dwarfism and arthrogryposis are at risk for postoperative respiratory arrest or obstruction due to intrinsic abnormalities of palatal and pharyngeal musculature.

Summary

Over the past 20 years, the innovations in spinal instrumentation pioneered by Harrington, Dwyer, Luque, and others have provided us with the means of managing all sorts of difficult and complex spinal deformities. With careful patient evaluation, close attention to indications, and careful preoperative planning, these techniques can be employed safely and effectively. The surgeon must be skilled in the use of these systems and must have an understanding of the various characteristics of the disorder that he is managing. The segmental spinal instrumentation system of Luque has rapidly evolved to a point at which stable fixation can be obtained in all but the most extreme circumstances. Undoubtedly, this system will continue to evolve to meet better the needs of the patient and his surgeon.

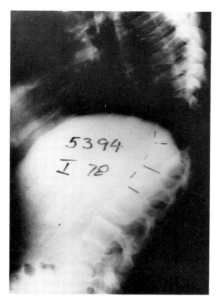

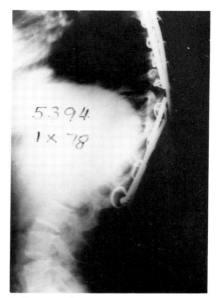

Fig. 4-10A. A 16-year-old patient with post-poliomyelitis sequelae with a collapsing curve, making a 47° thoracolumbar kyphosis.

B, Postoperative photo of SSI with Hibbs-Risser arthrodesis and pseudarthrosis at the thoracolumbar junction due to lack of adequate correction of the deformity.

Editor's Commentary

An especially important aspect of SSI is improving the lifestyle of the patient. There is nothing worse that being a spectator at the death by asphyxia of an untreated muscular dystrophy patient. It must be emphasized that in this type of problem I go even further than Dr. Herring in the prevention of spinal deformity. I believe that a child who sits in a tripod posture, using his arms for support, is a candidate for segmental rodding even if there is no structural curve (Fig. 4-9). This, together with hyperlordosis and a balanced curve, will ultimately free his hands and better his way of life.

SSI can and should be used to give structural support and advantageous sagittal curves. There are two words of warning, however:

1. Most of our instrument failures in this group of patients have come from not correcting a thoracolumbar kyphosis, which with two long lever arms will make a stress riser at this point (Fig. 4-10).

2. In introducing hyperlordosis, it is easy to narrow the AP diameter of the chest at the site of diaphragmatic insertion, in this way reducing the vital capacity of the

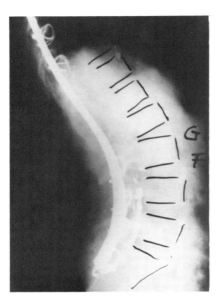

Fig. 4-11. Paraplegic 14-year-old male in whom too much hyperlordosis was introduced, with a corresponding loss of vital capacity.

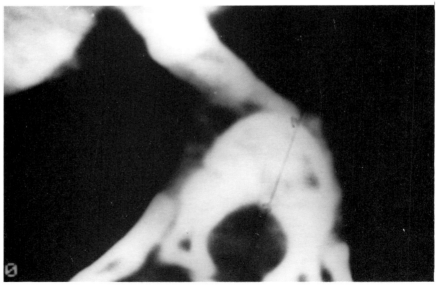

Fig. 4-12A. CAT scan of the apex of a juvenile idiopathic scoliotic curve with 28° of rotation.

patient and leaving him out of balance (Fig. 4-11). Recently, we have been using CAT scans to measure rotation, and we feel that this is the only true evaluation of apical rotation (Fig. 4-12). Short of total segmental mobility, we have failed in correcting this defect.

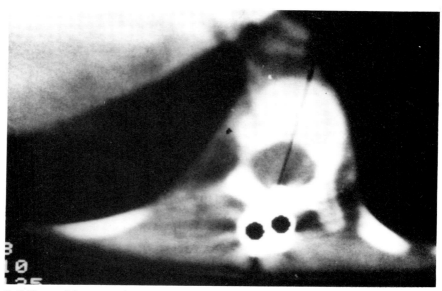

B, CAT scan of the same patient at the same vertebral level after SSI without arthrodesis, demonstrating no change in the rotatory deformity.

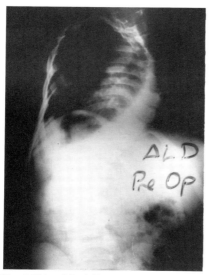
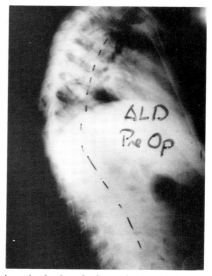

Fig. 4-13*A* and *B.* A 7-year-old male with Du-chenne's muscular dystrophy with a thoracic

hyperkyphosis and a thoracolumbar scoliosis of 85°. The structural thoracic curve is 70°.

In patients with severe deformities, we certainly agree that anterior and posterior procedures must be done. I would go even further than Dr. Herring, stating that multiple vertebrectomy procedures, especially in severe kyphosis or pelvic obliquity, provide shortening with a greater degree of safety than elongation

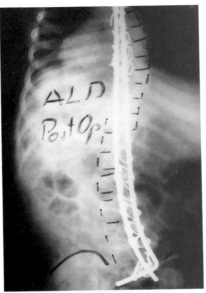

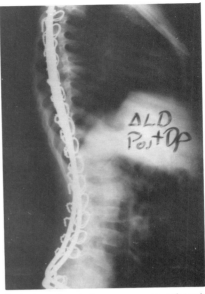

C and *D*. Correction of both curves below 25° with good AP head-over-pelvis balance. On the lateral x-rays, a total correction of the thoracolumbar kyphosis is seen, producing hyper-

lordosis and posterior compensatory thoracic kyphosis. These in turn produce a head-righting reflex.

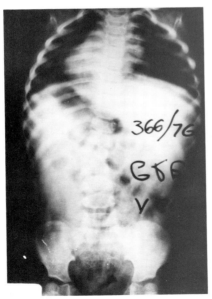

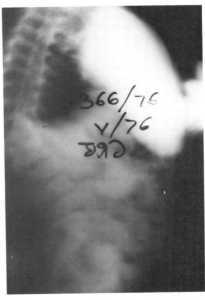

Fig. 4-14*A* and *B*. A congenital posterior, left lateral hemivertebra in a 3-year-old male, pro-

ducing a slightly unbalanced scoliosis from T11 to L2 and a severe kyphosis from T9 to T4.

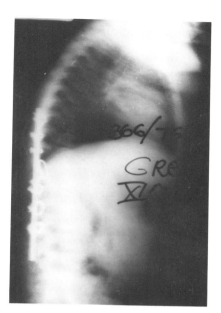

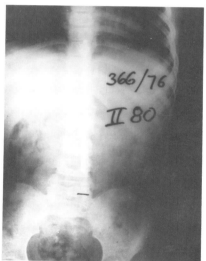

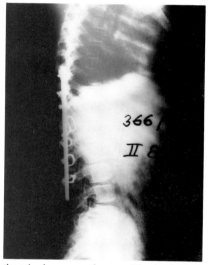

C, Same patient as Fig. 4-14*A* postoperatively, with a convex straight segmental rod from T9 to L4. Total correction of the kyphosis is seen.

D and *E,* Four-year follow-up x-ray of patient in Fig. 4-14*A.* In the AP position, there has been alignment of the growth centers to produce a straight spine in spite of the hemivertebra. There has been 2.6 cm of growth in the area of immobilization. In the lateral x-rays, growth is shown clearly by the fact that in the immediate postoperative picture, the end of the bar was at the L5-S1 level, and it was 3.3 cm to the most caudal wire. In the four-year follow-up picture, the spine has assumed a normal lumbar lordosis and thoracic kyphosis. The caudal end of the rod is now at the L4-L5 interspace, and the distance between the end of the rod and the immediate wire is only 2 cm, representing 1.3 cm of growth in seven segments in four years, which is expected. A straight AP spine has been obtained, correcting rotational deformity. A normal sagittal alignment is also evident.

carries. We normally do our final correction of these patients when they are completely awake and strapped down to the operating table. Five minutes after total correction is obtained, the patient is put back to sleep, and then he is awakened once again to recheck his neurologic status before leaving the operating room.

In severely paralyzed patients with a short life expectancy, we like to use SSI early without an arthrodesis. We have little worry about losing some growth potential. In our small series of twelve patients with an average follow-up of six years, with two rods we have only had one instrument failure, and the deformity produced has not necessitated a second intervention (Fig. 4-13). Not doing an arthrodesis in these patients obviously will reduce the surgical risk and blood loss. This is not possible in osteogenesis imperfecta, however. Our area of immobilization in these severely handicapped children is always very long and covers both AP and sagittal curves from beginning to end.

Application of SSI in congenital scoliosis has offered some interesting possibilities. There is no doubt that if operated on soon enough, the concave side of the intervertebral spaces can be opened, and with time they will fill in. There is also no question that these patients will grow in the area of immobilization. Our best results have been with a single convex rod (Fig. 4-14).

The Leatherman approach of extirpating the wedged vertebra anteriorly and then applying SSI fixation without arthrodesis in the back is mechanically sound, and it seems to be producing excellent results in his hands.

Again, I repeat, "Preventing deformity is the name of the game!"

References

1. Dwyer AF: Experience of anterior correction of scoliosis. Clin Ortho 93:191-206, 1973.

2. Gruca A: The pathogenesis and treatment of idiopathic scoliosis. J Bone Jt Surg 40A:570-584, 1958.

3. Harrington PR: Treatment of scoliosis. J Bone Jt Surg 44A:591-610, 1962.

4. Hibbs RA: An operation for progressive spinal deformities—A preliminary report of three cases from the service of the orthopaedic hospital. NY Med J 93:1013-1016, 1911.

5. Luque ER: The anatomic basis and development of segmental spinal instrumentation. Spine, Volume 7, Number 3:256-275, 1982.

6. Wenger DR, Carollo JJ, Wilkerson JA Jr: Biomechanics of scoliosis correction by segmental spinal instrumentation. Spine, Volume 7, Number 3:260-265, 1982.

7. Luque ER: Vertebral column transposition. Orthopaedic transactions. J Bone Jt Surg 7(1):29, 1983.

Preparation, Technique, and Personal Experience

5

Introduction

Segmental spinal instrumentation (SSI) with Luque rods has become an increasingly popular method for the surgical management of spinal disorders of various causes. After visiting Dr. Eduardo Luque in the early part of 1979 and learning his technique, this author shortly thereafter performed his first segmental spinal instrumentation for the stabilization of a fractured thoracic spine with paraplegia. Subsequently, the author's initial experience was gained in patients with neuromuscular spinal deformities and severe handicaps, many of whom would have either been denied treatment or been subject to an unacceptable high risk of postoperative complications if conventional means of internal fixation and postoperative immobilization were employed.[3] Confidence and experience with the technique in 107 patients to date, coupled with reproducible satisfactory results, have convinced this author that segmental spinal instrumentation is a worthwhile addition to the spinal surgeon's armamentarium. Furthermore, the

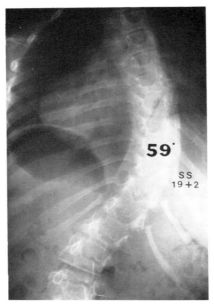 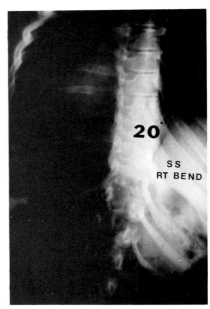

Fig. 5-1A. S.S., a 19-plus 2-year-old with spastic cerebral palsy and a long right thoracic scoliosis of 59 degrees without significant pelvic obliquity.

B, Flexibility on forced bending to 20 degrees.

technique is suitable for nearly all types of spinal deformity for which rigid internal fixation is necessary.[4-7]

This chapter presents this author's clinical indications for the use of SSI, describes the surgical technique used exclusively for the past two years, and discusses results, complications, and controversies associated with the system.

Clinical Indications

Neuromuscular Scoliosis

The management of spinal deformities in patients with neuromuscular disorders has always presented a challenge to the spinal surgeon. The severity of the deformity, respiratory compromise, weak bone stock for instrument fixation, and, in certain patients, mental retardation and seizure disorders have added to the difficulty of the task. Traditional methods of treatment, including Harrington rod instrumentation and posterior fusion alone or combined with anterior fusion, with

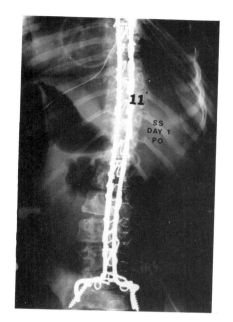

C, Correction to 11 degrees in the immediate postoperative period. Distal end rod configuration fashioned for anchoring over the sacral alae. Cancellous screws driven through S1 facets into the sacral alae anchor the laterally directed arms of the distal end to the alae. This configuration may be used when there is no pelvic obliquity or in kyphotic deformities when fusion to sacrum is necessary.

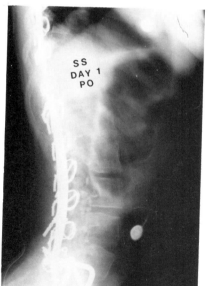

D, Distal end configuration in the lateral plane and preservation of sagittal curves.

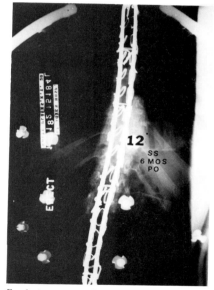

E, Anteroposterior x-ray six months postoperatively demonstrating proximal L configuration that fixes the construct distance, preventing slippage of wires over the proximal ends with increase in thoracic kyphosis. An early solid fusion is evident.

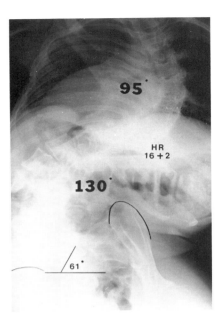

Fig. 5-2A. H.R., a 16-plus 2-year-old female with mental retardation and spastic cerebral palsy with a severe rigid, double-major scoliosis. Pelvic obliquity measures 61 degrees from the horizontal; right hip is subluxed.

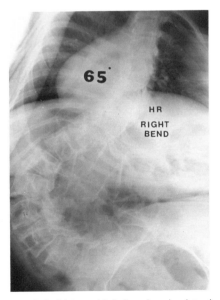

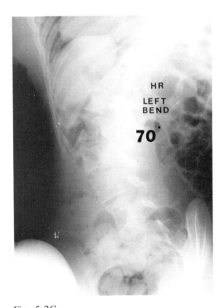

B and C. Right and left forced supine lateral bending demonstrates curve rigidity with correction to 65° and 70°, respectively.

Fig. 5-2C.

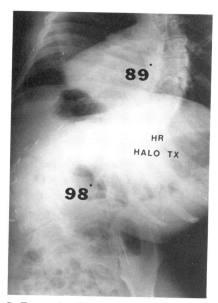

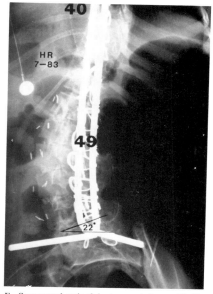

D, Two weeks after anterior release through a left thoracoabdominal approach and halo traction, correction of the curve occurred to 89° and 98°, respectively. Correction is much less than obtained by forced bending films. Halo traction serves only to stabilize the spine and allow the patient to attain the upright position.

E, Segmental spinal instrumentation with ¼-inch Luque rods anchored in the iliac wings. Correction of the curves to 40° and 49°, respectively. Pelvic obliquity was reduced to 22°. Spinal cord monitoring was employed.

or without the use of Dwyer instruments, have proven to be less than ideal.[8,9] The disadvantages of these techniques include: the tenuous fixation in osteoporotic bone, the necessity for cautious nursing techniques in the immediate postoperative period to prevent instrument dislodgement, less latitude in the application of respiratory care, the need for prolonged postoperative immobilization and careful handling, and delayed instrument failure secondary to pseudarthrosis.[8,10-12]

Patients with neuromuscular spinal deformities are ideal candidates for segmental spinal instrumentation for all the above reasons. Special attention must be given to the patient's deformity, however, before deciding on the ideal method or combination of methods to be used. The most straightforward deformity is flexible scoliosis with normal or near-normal sagittal curves. Passive correctable curves can undergo instrumentation and be aligned so that spinal fusion may proceed, particularly along axial stress lines (Fig. 5-1). Wenger et al, in a biomechanical analysis of scoliosis correction using segmental spinal instrumentation, has theorized that if scoliotic curves are reduced to less than 44 degrees, further correction and maintenance of this correction are best achieved with segmental spinal instrumentation.[13,14] Heeding Eduardo Luque's cautionary statement that curves should not be corrected beyond ten degrees of their maximal forced side-bending correc-

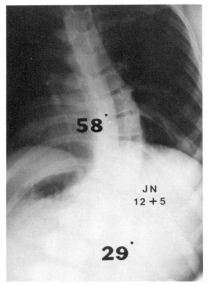

Fig. 5-3A. J.N., a 12-plus 5-year-old female with a 58° progressive, right thoracic idiopathic scoliosis.

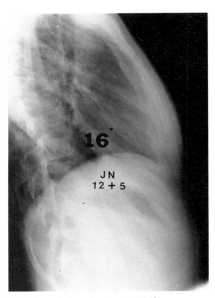

B, A thoracic hypokyphosis of 16°.

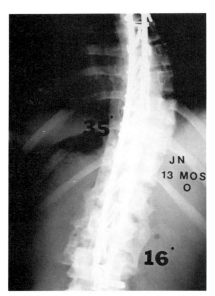

C, Thirteen months postoperatively, with correction of the right thoracic curve to 35°. A solid intertransverse process spinal fusion is noted throughout the entire curve that underwent instrumentation.

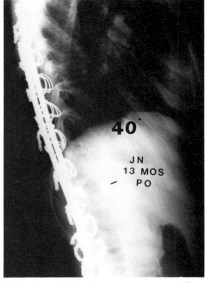

D, The thoracic hypokyphosis measures 40° on lateral x-rays 13 months postoperatively.

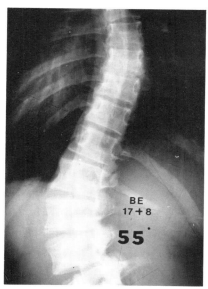

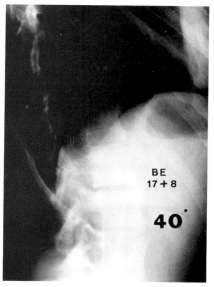

Fig. 5-4A. B.E., a 17-plus 8-year-old female with left lumbar idiopathic scoliosis.

B, Lateral x-ray shows lumbar lordosis to be 40°.

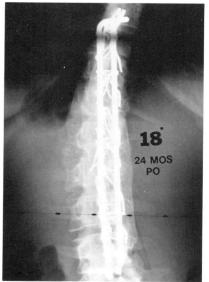

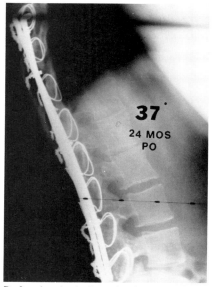

C, Anteroposterior film 24 months postoperatively shows a solid fusion radiographically, no wire loosening, and curve correction maintained at 18°.

D, Lumbar lordosis maintained at 37° 24 months postoperatively.

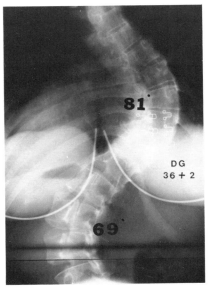

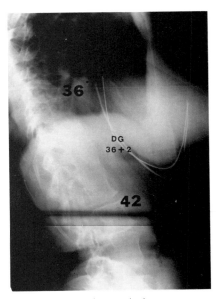

Fig. 5-5A. D.G., 36-plus 2-year-old female with severe, flexible, untreated right thoracic, left lumbar idiopathic scoliosis.

B, Lateral x-rays show sagittal curves to measure 36° and 42°, respectively.

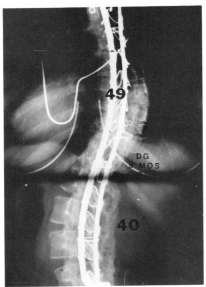

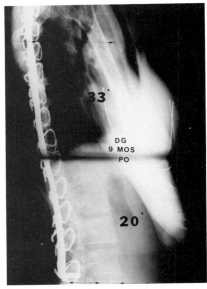

C, Anteroposterior x-ray nine months postoperatively showing satisfactory spinal fusion and correction of the double curves to 49° and 40°, respectively.

D, Lateral x-ray shows sagittal curves maintained in the physiologic range but reduced when compared with preoperative films. More sagittal contouring could have been applied to these rods.

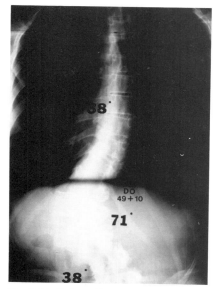

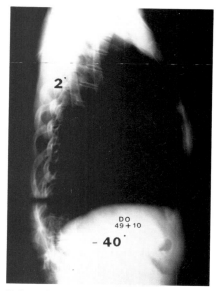

Fig. 5-6A. D.O., a 49-plus 10-year-old female with a severe, untreated, painful left lumbar scoliosis measuring 71°. Compensatory curves above and below measure 38°. Her trunk is markedly shortened, with ribs abutting against the pelvis.

B, Lateral x-rays show reversal of the normal sagittal curves with a 2° thoracic kyphosis and a minus 40° lumbar lordosis.

tion (to prevent neurologic compromise), we have routinely performed one-stage posterior instrumentation and fusion only if the lateral curvature can be corrected passively to 55 degrees or less.[6,7] If the curves are not passively correctable beyond this point, then they are felt to be rigid and require a two-stage procedure. This includes anterior diskectomy and release with anterior interbody fusion, followed by a two-to-three week period of Halo wheelchair traction or Halo-Cotrell traction. Then instrumentation is done posteriorly using segmental instruments and spinal fusion (Fig. 5-2). Failure to adhere to these time-tested principles will guarantee less success. If the lateral curvature is associated with kyphosis, or if kyphosis is present alone, the same considerations regarding flexibility apply.

It is this author's belief that almost all patients who are candidates for surgery can tolerate at least partial immobilization in the postoperative period with a light orthosis. A few patients who have severe respiratory compromise or no cutaneous sensation, or both, can be treated without postoperative immobilization, but the demands placed on their spines must be low.

Idiopathic Scoliosis

As experience was gained with the technique of segmental spinal instrumentation, patients with idiopathic scoliosis were considered candidates for segmental instru-

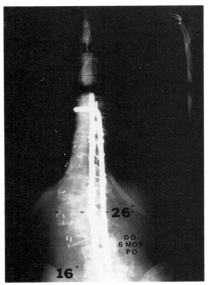 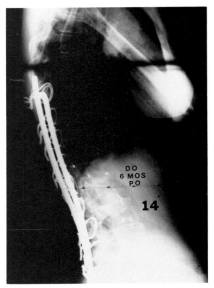

C, Because of curve rigidity, this patient underwent a two-stage procedure: an anterior thoracolumbar release followed by two weeks of halo traction and then posterior instrumentation with ¼-inch Luque rods. Six months postoperatively, her curves are maintained at 26° with reduction of the two compensatory curves to 10° and 16°, respectively. Her trunk was elongated sufficiently to bring her ribs several inches out of her pelvis.

D, Lateral x-ray six months postoperatively shows restoration of near-normal sagittal curves, with a 27° thoracic kyphosis and a 14° lumbar lordosis.

mentation. The author feels that for patients with idiopathic scoliosis, the absolute indications for SSI are to maintain and preserve, if not restore, sagittal contours to the postural curves. Therefore, patients with thoracic hypokyphosis or frank thoracic lordosis are ideal candidates, since the Harrington rod does little in the way of restoring a normal thoracic kyphosis (Fig. 5-3).[15,16] Moe and others have pointed out the importance of using a square-ended Harrington rod and of conforming the rod so as to lose as little lumbar lordosis as possible. Despite this, the inherent distraction forces of the Harrington rod tend to produce more flattened lumbar spines than normal curvatures. Therefore, the maintenance of postural lordosis would appear to be very important in the prevention of a flat back, especially in the patient who cannot compensate by increasing the lordosis below the level of the fusion (Fig. 5-4). These patients, as Moe pointed out, have pain not only in the upper thoracic and cervical area, but also in the knees and lower back, because of the forward thrust of the body.[17] Contouring of the L-rods permits a smooth transition between the fused segments of the lumbar spine and the remaining mobile segments, and perhaps in the future will prevent the increased incidence of low back pain, especially in those patients fused to L4.[18] In idiopathic scoliosis, the application of SSI is indicated in patients in whom a cast would represent either an emotional or a physical hardship. More often than not, the ever-increasing adult population seeking surgical treatment will tolerate a cast poorly for social, psychologic, and occupational reasons (Fig. 5-5). Occasionally in the adolescent age group, a cast is not feasible because of the same reasons. When rigid lateral curves and kyphosis are present, the same principles apply as for any spinal deformity. Correctability must be obtained with anterior procedures prior to the application of SSI (Fig. 5-6).

Patient Preparation and Monitoring

At New York Medical College, it is our routine preoperatively to evaluate all patients, with not only routine blood work and urinalysis but also pulmonary function testing, analysis of arterial blood gasses, and an automated physiologic hemodynamic profile obtained via the Swan-Ganz catheter. When intelligence and cooperation permit, patients with neuromuscular spinal deformity or severe respiratory compromise secondary to their scoliosis, or both, undergo intense preoperative respiratory preparation at home for at least a month prior to surgery, and occasionally in the hospital one week prior to surgery. This entails intense use of incentive spirometry and an intense course of intermittent positive-pressure breathing. Mentally retarded patients receive a course of chest physiotherapy and postural drainage prior to surgery. Respiratory techniques learned and applied prior to surgery are implemented immediately postoperatively, with early assumption of the erect position.

An ongoing study is currently in progress at New York Medical College in conjunction with the Department of Anaesthesiology and Departments of Pulmonary Medicine, in an attempt to correlate pulmonary function with data obtained from right heart Swan-Ganz catheterization. Preliminary results have clearly shown that an increase in the right ventricular stroke-work index is an indicator of increased right heart work in patients with idiopathic scoliosis. This change is present in patients who have normal pulmonary function and thoracic curves of less than 65 degrees. Further data are being collected in an attempt to correlate the degree of curvature and pulmonary function with data from right-heart catheterization. This correlation might then be utilized in patients with mental retardation, who are unable to cooperate with routine pulmonary function testing.[19]

For correction of scoliosis and kyphosis in rigid deformities, Halo-Cotrell or Halo wheelchair traction has been utilized in the interval between anterior and posterior surgery. It is the author's impression that Halo traction does not increase the ultimate correction, but serves the important function of stabilizing the spine and allowing the patient to be upright, out of bed in a wheelchair, or, if physically

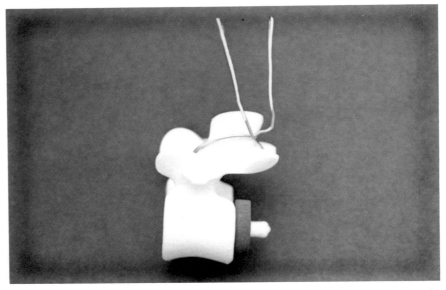

Fig. 5-7. Model illustrates method used by author to fix wire to lamina safely prior to rod placement in order to avoid accidental anterior displacement into the spinal canal with manipulation.

possible, ambulating with a modified wheelchair traction apparatus. The upright position has obvious benefits in the prevention of pulmonary, urinary, and vascular complications.

Surgical Technique

Patient positioning is of utmost importance in surgery. We have found the Wilson frame for average-sized patients, or chest rolls for small patients to be the surfaces of choice, offering the most adaptability in positioning. Ideally, positioning should allow the abdominal contents to fall anteriorly, to decrease venous bleeding and to so position the patient that his sagittal curves are as near normal as possible. Pelvic obliquity can be difficult to control, but positioning of the lower extremities, high side leg traction, or the use of a Harrington outrigger for distraction of the pelvis can aid in correction. Positioning is of utmost importance, since thoracic hypokyphosis and lumbar hyperlordosis both approximate the laminae, making exposure and removal of the ligamentum flavum much more difficult. Surgical exposure is carried out in a routine manner. After initial subperiosteal dissection of the paraspinous muscles, electrocautery is used to expose widely the posterior bony elements to the tips of the transverse processes in both the thoracic and the lumbar spine. In patients requiring fusion to the sacrum, the sacrum and iliac wings are exposed to the level of S2. Use of electrocautery in the exposure dramatically reduces blood loss and creates a clean, wide operative field. The remaining soft tissue is then meticulously removed with curettes and rongeurs in order to prepare a bed for a posterior intertransverse and facet fusion. With a metal marker in a spinous process, a posteroanterior x-ray is taken so that unnecessary dissection proximally—and especially distally—is not carried out. Great care is taken to preserve the joint capsules, the ligamentum flavum, and the interspinous ligament articulating with the first mobile segment at the lower end of the fusion. In the lumbar spine, the ligamentum flavum is easily removed by using a three-millimeter Leksell rongeur to take an initial midline bite. One bite usually exposes the epidural fat. Then, using a straight or gently angled one-millimeter Leksell rongeur, the flavum is removed laterally on either side of the midline to the facets. A piece of gelfoam is then placed over the epidural fat. In the thoracic spine, many patients have long, narrow spinous processes which overlap, completely obscuring the ligamentum flavum. These spinous processes must be cut with a rongeur, and angled in such a way as to leave a protruding bit against which the rods may abut. The ligamentum flavum may then be removed in the same manner as in the lumbar spine. Except in the tightest circumstances, using three-millimeter and one-millimeter Leksell rongeurs for ligamentum flavum removal has been found to be a safe and quick means of exposure of the epidural space. Occasional bleeding of epidural veins can occur, but, with care, this can be minimized. In our experience, we have had no dural lacerations. Patients with Scheuermann's kyphosis or severe hypokyphosis, and adult patients with severe scoliosis can present a greater challenge in ligamentum flavum removal. In patients with Scheuermann's kyphosis, we have noted that the thoracic facets appear to be overgrown medially and, in some cases, almost touching—leaving a minimal remnant of ligamentum flavum. In patients with severe hypokyphosis, the shingling effect of the thoracic vertebrae is so great that the ligamentum flavum is almost absent. Severe lateral curvatures have a distorted configuration on the concavity, with shortened and abutting laminae. In these instances, removing bone to allow room for adequate wire passage is more tedious but must be performed adequately. The facets in both the thoracic and the lumbar spine are then removed with a three-millimeter Leksell rongeur, in preparation for a facet fusion. Occasionally, thoracic facets are obliterated according to the method of Moe, using a straight Cobb gouge.[20] Cortical cancellous bone is harvested in a routine fashion from the iliac crest, and plugs of cancellous bone are then meticulously impacted bilaterally into all the lumbar facets to be fused, and into the concave thoracic facets. We fuse the lumbar facets bilaterally, where spinal fusion is usually more difficult to obtain. We have found it necessary to fuse only the concave side of the thoracic curve, leaving the convex facets free to approximate with correction. Facet removal and facet fusion are performed prior to wire passage. Thus, there is minimal manipulation and insertion of instruments in the field after sublaminar wires have been passed.

For the past two years, it has been our practice to pass bilateral doubled 18-

gauge wires over the entire length of the instrumented curve, except at the proximal and distal vertebrae, where bilateral doubled 16-gauge wires are used. We have found this to be quicker and safer in the long run than cutting and manipulating cut wires from side to side. Furthermore, wires fabricated with the soldered ball ends have no sharp points projecting to snag an operator's glove. All wires are passed distally to proximally and pulled to even lengths on either side of the lamina. The proximal end is bent distally over the superior edge of the lamina and kept toward the midline, with its end protruding out of the field (Fig. 5-7). This serves two functions: (1) It provides a margin of safety in case of an accidental push of the wire tips in the direction of the spinal canal. The wires, so bent, cannot be plunged into the neural tissues. (2) Furthermore, it orients the wires so that the rods may be easily laid down between the proximal and distal wire ends, without having to be untwisted or further manipulated.[21] Fingertip control is stressed, and a long needle holder is used in handling and passing wires. If the spine is to undergo instrumentation to the sacrum, double 16-gauge wires are passed through the first posterior sacral foramen out through the L5-S1 interspace. This is felt to aid in fixation of the rod to the sacrum. Holes are then made in the iliac crests, using a curved awl or a flexible 3/16-inch drill. In this instance, harvesting of the iliac crest is performed in such a way as to leave a bicortical square of bone in the area where the L portion of the rod would protrude. The 90-degree L's normally must be fashioned by the surgeon, using tubular rod benders. It is our practice to place a gentle anterior bend at the tip of the L, to reduce the direct lateral protrusion of the tip into the gluteal soft tissues.

Wire passage at the distal vertebrae deserves special consideration, since it is our belief that the interspinous ligament, ligamentum flavum, and facet joints and capsules should be preserved in their entirety, so that the mechanics of this first mobile motion segment are disturbed as little as possible. To accomplish this, the paraspinous muscles are subperiosteally elevated away from the interspace, exposing the ligamentum flavum and interspinous ligament. An angled No. 2 curette is then used to skive the ligamentum flavum off the undersurface of the last lamina to undergo instrumentation. In this manner, a small hole is made between the ligamentum flavum anteriorly and the inferior portion of the lamina posteriorly for passage of the double 16-gauge wire. Care must be taken to detach the entire ligamentum flavum from the undersurface of the lamina, so that wire passage can be accomplished gently. A drill hole is then made in this last spinous process.

Initially, it was our practice to fashion a preoperative template from the forced bending films out of a malleable rod. With experience, we have abandoned this, and we now contour the rods on the operating table, using the x-rays and the anatomic preparation in the operating room. Compensatory curves must be built into the rods in order that proximal and distal ends will be in plumb. This insures compensation of the corrected spine.

As mentioned previously, care is taken in rigid spines not to exceed 10 degrees of correction, using the preoperative forced bending films as a point of reference. Kyphosis and lordosis are then prebent into the rods, using a French rod bender. Depending on the patient's size, either 3/16-inch or quarter-inch rods are selected.

Handling 3/16-inch rods is easier, and because of their greater flexibility, overcorrection is probably impossible, since the rod bends when the spine reaches its limits of elasticity. The rods are generally inserted applying the concave rod first. Care must be taken at both proximal and distal ends that the L-portion is lying over bony lamina and not in the interspace, where it could rotate anteriorly and cause neural damage. The rod is easily laid down between bent wires, keeping the soldered ends laterally and the hairpin ends medially. In this way, much of the confusion of "look-alike" cut ends is eliminated. The wires are twisted clockwise with fingertip and needle-holder manipulation and then tightened with a safety wire twister, first tightening those wires at the proximal and distal ends, where the rod lies closest to the posterior elements.

With long instruments, counterforces are applied over the apex of the curve and to the rod, so that the rod and spine are approximated and the stresses are relieved from the wire and wire-bone interface. This is most important along the concavity of the curve, where the rod is most displaced from the posterior elements. In like fashion, the convex rod is inserted, and wire tightening is begun proximally. Then again, using counterforces against rod and spine, the distal end is approximated to the posterior elements. Lane bone clamps are then applied to the rods to approximate slowly those areas that are still separated. Sixteen-gauge coupling wires are then applied at the proximal and distal ends and to the middle of the rod. Further tightening of any loose wires is carried out, and the wires are cut, leaving one centimeter protruding. These protruding ends are bent distally so that they lie over the rod and are flat on the posterior surface of the rod. This leaves all the metal in one area, without wire tips protruding haphazardly. This facilitates decortication lateral to the rods and the placement of the bone graft. It also facilitates reexposure if rod removal or repair of pseudarthrosis, or both, is necessary at a later date.

Spinal fusion is then performed in a meticulous fashion, decorticating all the transverse processes in both the thoracic and lumbar spines and applying autogenous bone bilaterally in the lumbar spine, bilaterally over the proximal two segments in the thoracic spine, and over the entire concavity in the thoracic spine. If there is sufficient bone remaining, this may be applied to the convexity in the thoracic spine. In patients with normal pelvic configuration, a graft from one iliac crest has been found to be sufficient. In many patients with neuromuscular scoliosis, even bilateral iliac grafts may prove to be insufficient, and supplemental homologous bank bone can be used. Closure over subcutaneous hemovac drainage is performed in the usual fashion.

Postoperative Management

All patients are mobilized as soon as pain permits. On the second day, patients are allowed to sit in bed, inclined forty to forty-five degrees, if vital signs are stable.

TABLE 5-1.
Patient Data—Neuromuscular Scoliosis

| | | | | | PREOPERATIVE CURVES† | | | | Correct S/K/L | Pelvic Obliquity | DECOMPENSATION‡ | | Level |
Pt	Age	Sex	Dx	FU*	Scoliosis	Kyphosis	Lordosis	Bend	Init Final	Preop Final	Head Preop Final	Trunk Preop Final	Fused
1	17	M	MD	21	T5-L5=93			49°	39°/58°	30°/15°	4.3/4.6	8/4	T5-S2
2	18	M	TP	19	T9-L4=103			90°	70°/90°	34°/38°	0/2.6	13/9.6	T2-S2
3	15	M	FA	dec	T5-L3=102			47°	43°/dec	7°/dec	9.1/dec	11.5/dec	T5-S2
4	7	F	MM	15	T5-T11=30		T8-L5=90	L75°	S23°/28° L35°/40°	15°/3°	4.4/1.2	4.9/2.5	T9-S2
5	17	M	CP MR	15	T6-L3=45			5°	20°/26°	2°/0°	0.6/0.9	5.6/3.7	T5-S2
6	18	M	CP MR	15	T3-T11=38 T11-L5=45	T7-L3=62		S10° S2° K12°	S15°/19° S2°/12° K31°/36° L21°/26°	12°/2°	5.4/1.8	6.6/3.1	T3-S2
7	16	M	MD	14	T1-T7=40 T7-L5=76			48°	28°/28° 37°/42°	17°/2°	6.3/4.3	5.7/1.9	T3-S2
8	16	M	CP MR	10	T10-L3=37	T1-L3=140		S3° K45°	S0°/0° K32°/59° L29°/30°	20°/6°	2.6/6	5.9/2.6	T2-S2
9	16	F	CP MR	10	T2-L2=80			22°	26°/35°	6°/7°	1.5/−1.2	9.7/3.8	T2-S2
10	16	M	VG	10	T6-L3=65		L1-L5=88 T1-L5=145	S48° L42°	S28°/26° L35°/36°	15°/5°	2.6/2.1	7.4/3.1	T2-S2

TABLE 5-1.
Patient Data (continued) Neuromuscular Scoliosis

Pt	Age	Sex	Dx	FU*	PREOPERATIVE CURVES†					Pelvic Obliquity Preop Final	DECOMPENSATION‡		Level Fused
					Scoliosis	Kyphosis	Lordosis	Bend	Correct S/K/L Init Final		Head Preop Final	Trunk Preop Final	
11	29	F	FA	9	T4-T12=92 T12-L5=61	T1-T12=−51		59° 20°	K4°/13° 49°/57° 30°/37°	0°/0°	6.9/5	13.3/7.9	T2-S2
12	21	F	CP MR	9	T8-L4=85	T2-L2=98	L2-L5=50	S38° K55°	S31°/35° K50°/70° L31°/34°	41°/17°	1.7/−2	12/4.7	T2-S2
13	11	F	SMA	8	T6-L5=68			5°	8°/11°	22°/6°	1.5/1.5	9.4/1.7	T2-S2
14	20	F	CP MR	7	T10-L5=96	T3-L5=146		S30° K60°	S40°/42° K45°/62° L38°/41°	21°/9°	5.6/7.5	5.6/1.1	T1-S2
15	10	F	CN	4	T1-T9=48 T9-L5=80	T5-L4=67		S19° S32° K10°	S18°/21° S32°/38° K38°/41° L30°/39°	18°/8°	0.4/0.4	8.1/4.2	T3-S2
16	17	M	CP MR	2	T3-T10=25 T10-L4=55			20° 25°	22°/20° 19°/22°	11°/6°	1.8/−0.7	4.2/1.7	T4-S2
17	9	M	SMA	2	T6-L4=60	T3-L4=58		S5° K17°	S15°/17° K25°/25° L25°/25°	16°/2°	1/2	6.1/0	T2-S2

*in months.
†in degrees.
‡in centimeters.

TABLE 5-2.

Pre- and Postoperative Correction—Neuromuscular Scoliosis

	Preop Ave	(Range)	Bending Ave	(Range)	Degrees of Corr	% Corr	Initial Postop Curve	(Range)
Scoliosis	68°	(30°/103°)	29.3°	(3°/90°)	38.7°	56.9%	24.6°	(0/70°)
Kyphosis	95°	(58°/146°)	33.1°	(10°/60°)	61.9°	65.1%	36.3°	(25°/50°)
Lordosis	117°	(90°/145°)	63.5°	(42°/75°)	53.5°	45.7%	35°	(35°)
Pelvic Obliquity	18°	(6°/41°)	—	—	—	—	—	—
Head Decompensation	2.9cm	(0/9.1cm)	—	—	—	—	—	—
Trunk Shift	7.8cm	(4.2/13.3cm)	—	—	—	—	—	—

TABLE 5-2.
(Continued) Neuromuscular Scoliosis

	Degrees of Corr	% Corr	Final Curve	(Range)	Degrees of Corr	% Corr	Ave Corr Loss	% Loss
Scoliosis	43.4°	63.8%	32.5°	(0°/90°)	35.5°	52.2%	7.9°	11.6%
Kyphosis	58.7°	61.7%	48.8°	(25°/70°)	46.2°	48.6%	12.5°	13.1%
Lordosis	82°	70%	38°	(36°/40°)	79°	67.5%	3°	2.5%
Pelvic Obliquity	—	—	7.8°	(2°/38°)	10.2°	56.6%	—	—
Head Decompensation	—	—	2.2cm	(-1.2cm/7.5cm)	0.7cm	24.1%	—	—
Trunk Shift	—	—	3.5cm	(0cm/9.6cm)	4.3cm	55.1%	—	—

Between the third and fifth day, pain permitting, they may dangle at the bedside or sit in a chair. At this juncture, ambulatory patients are assisted with walking around the room, while a postoperative TLSO (thoracolumbar sacral orthosis) is fabricated. Nonambulatory patients are moved about in wheelchairs. In these patients, all that is necessary in the postoperative period is a Florida-type Jewett Hyperextension orthosis. All orthoses are worn only while the patient is upright and are removed for bathing and sleeping. Only occasionally have we had patients who would not tolerate any immobilization. These patients were usually nonambulators with severe pulmonary restriction or insensitive skin. With careful handling, no problems have occurred in these few patients.

Treatment Results

Neuromuscular Spinal Deformities

To date, 53 patients with neuromuscular scoliosis have undergone treatment with segmental spinal instrumentation and fusion. Forty-one had flexible curves and underwent one-stage procedures. Twelve had rigid curves and required anterior release and fusion, followed by Halo traction. Posterior segmental instrumentation and fusion were then done.

In an early review of 17 patients with neuromuscular spinal deformities operated on between 1979 and 1980, the longest follow-up was twenty-one months.[3] The underlying neurologic disorders were cerebral palsy, Duchenne's muscular dystrophy, Friedreich's ataxia, spinal muscular atrophy, congenital neuropathy and myelodysplasia, traumatic paraplegia, and von Gierke's disease. Seven of the seventeen patients had some degree of mental retardation, and all patients were restricted to a wheelchair both pre- and postoperatively. There were ten males and seven females. No patients had preoperative traction, and all had flexible curves, undergoing segmental spinal instrumentation and posterior fusion to the sacrum. The grafting material was autogenous bone graft in all patients. Spinal deformities were complex, six having severe kyphoscoliosis and two having severe lordoscoliosis. Preoperative scoliosis averaged 68 degrees (range: 30° to 103°). Preoperative kyphosis averaged 95 degrees (range: 58° to 146°), and preoperative lordosis averaged 117 degrees (range: 90° to 145°). Pelvic obliquity was present in 16 patients and averaged 18 degrees, with a range of 6 to 41 degrees.

Although these patients represented a group at high risk to develop pulmonary complications postoperatively, all but one were extubated within 72 hours. Tracheostomy was necessary in this one patient after ten days of intubation. There was one death in this early series in a patient with Friedreich's ataxia, who died of intractable congestive heart failure and pulmonary edema 36 hours after surgery. Twelve of these 17 patients were immobilized in TLSOs postoperatively, which were worn only when upright. Sixteen of the 17 patients returned to their preoperative ambulatory status. Fifteen demonstrated better sitting balance and

TABLE 5-3

Operative Data—Neuromuscular Scoliosis*

	Ave	(Range)	Level Fused
Operative Time	4'23"	(3'20"/5'15")	16.6 min/level
Anaesthetic Time	5'41"	(4'30"/7'20")	20.1 min/level
Estimated Blood Loss	2311cc	(1000/4000cc)	146.3cc/level

*Average no. of levels fused: 15.8 (Range: 10/18).

TABLE 5-4

Comparison of Immobilization in Idiopathic Scoliosis

	Curve	No.	Ave. Preop
Group I			
	T	7	57°
	TL	1	60°
	L	2	48°
	D	5	57°/48°
Group II			
	T	7	54°
	TL	1	40°
	L	1	40°
	D	3	56°/51°

increased sitting endurance, according to the people who cared for them. Daily hygiene and handling were also reported to be improved. One patient continued to have difficulty with trunk balance, sitting, and skin pressure. Further seating modifications had to be made in an attempt to equalize ischial weight distribution. This patient had a rigid spine, which was only minimally correctable passively. He should have undergone two-stage anterior and posterior surgery, instead of just a single-stage intervention. He was considered a failure of surgical treatment.

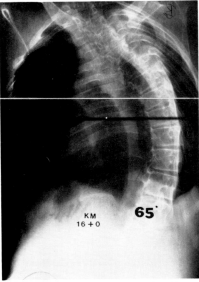

Fig. 5-8A. K.R., a 16-year-old male with von Gierke's disease and a long right thoracolumbar scoliosis of 65°.

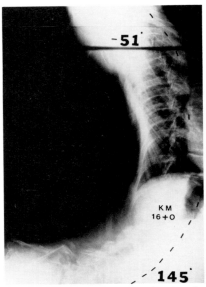

B, Sitting lateral x-rays show a continuation of a severe 145° lumbar lordosis into the thoracic spine, producing a minus 51° thoracic lordosis with marked reduction of the rib cage's antero-posterior diameter.

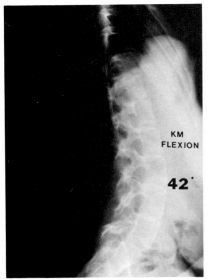

C, Forced flexion produced correction of the lordosis to 42°.

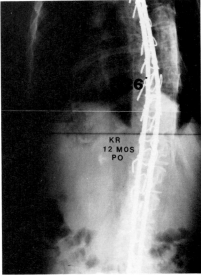

D, Twelve months postoperatively, correction is maintained at 26° despite loss of fixation of the upper two wires owing to distal migration of the rods.

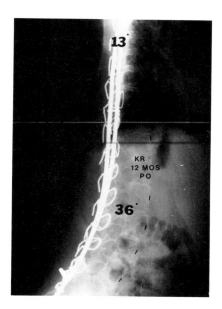

E, Lateral x-ray 12 months postoperatively shows restoration of sagittal curves and an increase in the chest's anteroposterior diameter.

Tables 5-1, 5-2, and 5-3 represent patient data from this preliminary study.

The average overall correction of lateral curvature as demonstrated on the initial erect radiograph was 63.8%. This deteriorated to 52.2%, with 11.6% loss over the follow-up period. The average loss of correction was 7.9°. Multiple upper-wire fatigue was felt to be reason for the resultant loss of instrumentation purchase in only one patient. In this patient, the loss was way above the average.

The average correction of kyphosis was 61.7% but deteriorated at follow-up by 13.1%. This was due to slipping of the wires over the rod ends at the uppermost vertebra. Since recognition of this problem, an L has been bent at the proximal end of one rod to stabilize the length of the corrected vertebral column. In one patient (Table 5-1, patient 12), loss of correction was thought to be due to the flexibility of the 3/16-inch rods. Therefore, the use of the more rigid quarter-inch rods is recommended when correcting kyphosis. In retrospect, perhaps the other two patients (8 and 14) would have lost less correction if a first-stage anterior release had been performed. In the six patients (6, 8, 12, 14, 15, and 17) who had pathologic kyphosis in the thoracic and lumbar spine, sagittal contouring of the Luque rod resulted in balanced postural curves with correction of the kyphosis and production of lumbar lordosis where it was previously nonexistent.

Pathologic lordosis was present in two patients in this series (4 and 10). Sagittal contouring of the rods allowed not only dramatic correction of lordosis, but also production of a balanced thoracic kyphosis. The average lordosis as demonstrated on initial upright film was 35 degrees, corrected from 117 degrees preoperatively. Only a 2.5% loss occurred over the follow-up period (Fig. 5-8).

Pelvic obliquity was corrected 65% (omitting patient 2, who should have had an anterior release and who lost pelvic fixation because of his curve rigidity). Without a distraction component in the segmental instrumentation system, pelvic obliquity is a difficult parameter to control. Patient positioning, high-side leg traction, or the use of a Harrington outrigger for distraction of the pelvic obliquity is available to obtain a more level pelvis.

Cephalopelvic decompensation, measured in centimeters as a deviation of the seventh cervical vertebra from a perpendicular line drawn through the center of the sacrum, averaged 2.9 centimeters preoperatively and 2.2 centimeters postoperatively. Final correction was only 24%. Trunk shift, measured in centimeters as deviation of the apical vertebrae from the cervicosacral perpendicular line, averaged 7.8 centimeters preoperatively and 3.5 centimeters postoperatively, with a correction of 55%. The less-than-ideal correction of cephalopelvic decompensation was felt to be due to several factors: (1) failure to fuse high enough into the thoracic spine in the early patients in this series; (2) failure to contour enough compensatory curve into the proximal end of the rods; and (3) fatigue or loss of purchase of the upper wires in several patients.

Complications

There was one death (patient 3)—a 15-year-old male with Friedreich's ataxia and cardiomyopathy. He died approximately 36 hours postoperatively secondary to intractable congestive heart failure and acute renal failure. There were five patients (1, 2, 8, 10, 14) who experienced some form of instrument failure. In patients 2, 8, and 14, this was thought to be responsible for the loss of correction that occurred. For example, patient 2, an 18-year-old male with traumatic paraplegia and very rigid scoliosis, was considered to have a poor result. His preoperative scoliosis measured 103° and corrected to only 90° on forced bending. The first erect postoperative radiograph showed correction of 70°. One month later, the curve measured 90° and remained at this magnitude at 19-month follow-up. Several wires had fatigued at the superior portion of the curve, with displacement of the rods to the convexity. His preoperative pelvic obliquity was 34° with a 13-cm trunk shift. At follow-up, his pelvic obliquity measured 38° with a 9.6-cm trunk shift. He was considered to be a failure of treatment, since the reason for his surgery was to level his pelvis and equalize pressure over the ischial tuberosities. This was not accomplished. An error in selection of this patient for segmental spinal instrumentation was made, since his curve was not flexible enough to allow satisfactory correction with a posterior procedure alone. The time-tested principles of spinal deformity surgery should have been applied to this patient, and correctability should have been gained with the use of combined anterior and posterior surgery (Fig. 5-9).

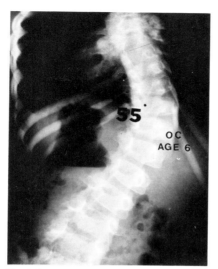

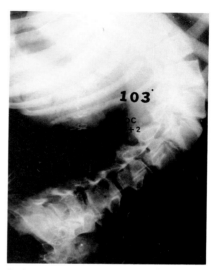

Fig. 5-9A. O.C. at age six, two years after traumatic paraplegia secondary to a fracture-dislocation of T5-T6. Note the fracture callus. A 55° right thoracolumbar paralytic scoliosis is evident at age 6.

B, At age 18, after urinary diversion and bilateral hip disarticulations during the intervening years, scoliosis had progressed to 103°.

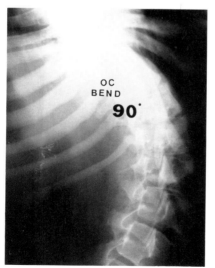

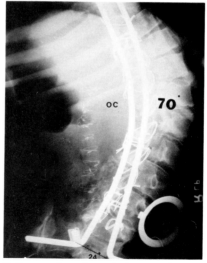

C, Forced bending demonstrates rigidity with correction to only 90°.

D, One month postoperatively, correction was 70° with reduction of severe pelvic obliquity to 24°. Four months postoperatively, pelvic obliquity had increased to 34° with loss of upper wire purchase and increase in the curvature to 90°. This patient should have had a two-stage anterior-posterior operation.

Patient 4, a seven-year-old with myelodysplasia, underwent a local procedure to trim a protruding wire at the distal end of the instrumentation one month postoperatively. This was successful, with no further complications and healing of a sinus tract.

Patient 8, a 16-year-old mentally retarded male with cerebral palsy and kyphoscoliosis, contracted aspiration pneumonia secondary to gastroesophageal reflux. This necessitated a fundoplication, gastrostomy, and tracheostomy. Since the experience with this patient, a barium-swallow esophagogram for all mentally retarded patients has become routine to ascertain the competency of their gastroesophageal junction. If it is incompetent preoperatively, straightening the spine and thus elongation of the intraabdominal structures will exacerbate the reflux. Therefore, it is recommended that a fundoplication and gastrostomy be performed prior to planned corrective spinal surgery.

In this initial group of 17 patients, operative time averaged four hours and 23 minutes. After gaining more experience with the technique, we have operated on the latter patients in our series over the past two years within three-and-one-half hours. Blood loss has remained fairly constant—between 1800 and 2500 ml (Table 5-3).

In the total series of 53 patients with neuromuscular scoliosis, two patients sustained deep-seated postoperative infections. Both patients were myelodysplastics with urinary diversions, in whom autologous bone for spinal fusion was supplemented by homologous bank bone. Debridement and irrigation without instrument removal was the treatment performed in these patients, with resultant wound closure by secondary intention. Their hospital course was protracted, and intravenous antibiotics were necessary.

Neurologic complications occurred in two patients in this population. One patient was a 16-year-old female with spastic diplegia and mental retardation who, in the immediate postoperative period, was felt to be neurologically intact. Shortly thereafter, a continuous clinical picture of "grand mal" seizures intermittently for 24 hours made neurologic assessment difficult. Once the patient's sensorium had returned to normal, she was discovered to have Brown-Séquard syndrome with mixed motor and sensory deficits. The segmental instruments and wires were removed, and the patient has made little recovery to date.

The second patient was a 14-year-old female with spastic athetoid cerebral palsy. During intraoperative correction, spinal-evoked potentials remained unchanged. This patient awoke with a motor deficit in the distribution of the right femoral nerve, however. Over a six-week period, she made a complete recovery. Patients with preexisting neuromuscular disorders, with or without mental retardation, are a difficult group of patients in which to detect motor or sensory deficits— and certainly minor paresthesias and root damage might go unnoticed in the postoperative period.

Three pseudarthroses have definitely been discovered in this group of patients, with multiple wire failure at the distal end in two and failure in the proximal end in one. One patient with spinal muscular atrophy underwent repair of a distal pseudarthrosis and replacement of fatigued wires, and has a resultant solid fusion.

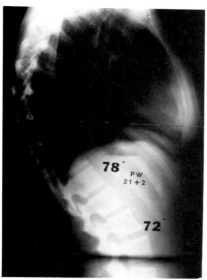

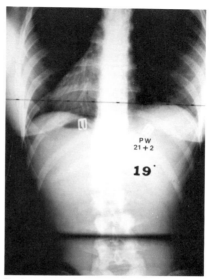

Fig. 5-10A. P.W., a 21-plus 2-year-old female with painful Scheuermann's kyphosis accompanied by compensatory hyperlordosis.

B, Anteroposterior x-ray shows minimal left thoracolumbar scoliosis.

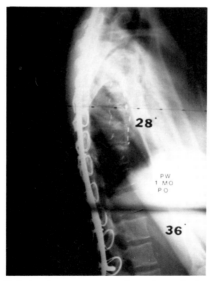

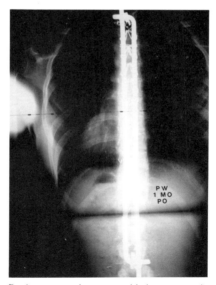

C, Lateral x-ray one month postoperatively shows maintenance of kyphosis correction to 28° and reduction of hyperlordosis to 36°. Instruments appear intact.

D, Anteroposterior x-ray with instruments in good position. At approximately two months postoperatively, the patient fell while wearing her brace. The three-month postoperative x-ray showed wire failure at the distal vertebra.

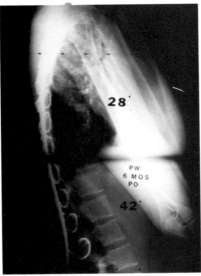

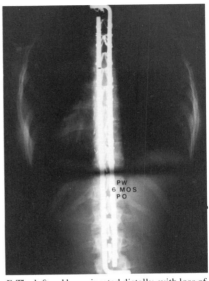

E, Lateral x-ray six months postoperatively shows fracture of the wires around the L2 vertebra with maintenance of kyphosis correction of 28°.

F, The left rod has migrated distally, with loss of purchase not only at the fractured wire site but also proximally. Further mobilization is indicated, and rod revision will be necessary in the future.

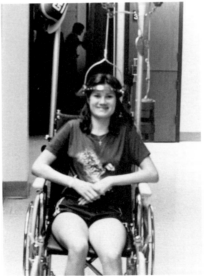

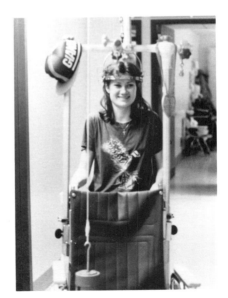

G, H, and *I,* Halo wheelchair traction between anterior and posterior surgery allowed this active patient to have exercise ambulation while in traction.

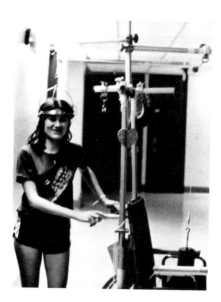

The second patient, with scoliosis secondary to a spinal cord injury, has refused further surgical intervention and, although the curve has deteriorated, is asymptomatic to date. The third patient, with spastic cerebral palsy, is under continued observation, has demonstrated no loss of correction, and is asymptomatic.

Scheuermann's Kyphosis

Patients with Scheuermann's kyphosis in whom brace treatment has failed or in whom diagnosis was delayed until after skeletal maturity are candidates for segmental instrumentation if their deformities are greater than 65 degrees. Over the past two years, four patients, all with pain and deformity, have been operated on. The principles outlined by Bradford are closely followed.[22] All patients had anterior diskectomies and interbody fusion over at least five vertebral levels through a thoracotomy approach. They were placed in Halo traction for two weeks and then underwent instrumentation and fusion with Luque rods, from at least T2 proximally to two levels below the distal end vertebra of the kyphosis. There were four patients in this small group, with an average age of 20 years. Follow-up was 17 months, with a range of six to 24 months. The average preoperative curve was 92 degrees, immediately postoperatively corrected to 38 degrees. At last follow-up film, correction had been lost to 44 degrees. The average estimated blood loss for the posterior procedure was 1575 ml.

Mechanical forces inherent in double-L rod insertion are ideal for the correction of kyphosis. Briefly, the technique involves securing one rod to the proximal arm of the kyphosis and the second rod to the distal arm. Slowly approximating the free ends, while sequentially tightening the sublaminar wires until the rods are secure, corrects the deformity.[16] The forces of correction are powerful and safe, since the spinal canal is shortened as correction takes place. Sublaminar passage enjoys a wide margin of safety, since the spinal cord is displaced anteriorly against the posterior aspect of the vertebral bodies. No neurologic complications or infections occurred in this group. In one patient, however, a 21-year-old female with a 78-degree kyphosis corrected to 28 degrees, two distal wires in the lamina of L2 fatigued, and purchase was lost (Fig. 5-10). No loss of the measured kyphosis between T3 and T12 was observed. At six months' follow-up, the fusion was proceeding satisfactorily. With loss of distal vertebra purchase, the rod migrated distally, losing contact with the proximal sublaminar wire. This sort of rod migration has been noted to a much lesser extent in several patients with scoliosis and is discussed later in this chapter. All patients with Scheuermann's kyphosis have been immobilized nine months postoperatively in a TLSO, with removal of the orthosis for bathing and sleeping. Satisfactory relief of pain and cosmetic improvement were achieved in all four patients. The average six-degree loss of correction over time was clinically insignificant. Further follow-up is needed in this group, however.

Idiopathic Curves

The surgical treatment of idiopathic scoliosis with segmental spinal instrumentation is surrounded by controversy. As with any new technique, safety and dexterity in its application, with careful attention to detail, are paramount to its success. Only after its use became routine in the most difficult of spinal deformities did this author attempt to apply it to the management of idiopathic scoliosis.

After retrospective analysis, a set of indications has evolved, based on the advantages that the segmental instrumentation system offers over Harrington instrumentation.[15] Absolute indications in the management of idiopathic scoliosis apply when restoration or preservation of physiologic postural curves is necessary. This is most important if thoracic scoliosis is accompanied by hypokyphosis or frank thoracic lordosis to prevent and improve further deterioration in pulmonary function.[23] Furthermore, when instrumentation is carried down low into the lumbar spine, the capability to contour normal sagittal curves into the rods allows preservation of normal lumbar lordosis with, theoretically, less compensatory hyperlordosis of the lower unfused lumbar segments. In terms of relative indications, we feel that when cast immobilization represents a social, psychologic, or occupational hardship, as may be present with many adult patients, its application deserves serious consideration.

Over a period of two years, 44 patients with idiopathic scoliosis were operated on. The average follow-up was 12.5 months, with a range of one to 27 months. There were 37 females and 7 males. The group was composed of 28 adolescents and 16 adults, whose average ages were 13.2 years and 35.6 years, respectively.

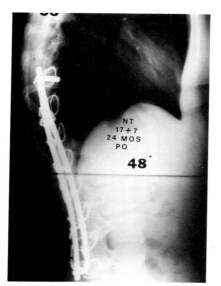 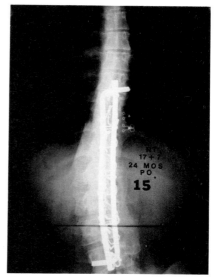

Fig. 5-11A and B. Distal wire failure in a 17-year-old female with left lumbar idiopathic scoliosis 24 months postoperatively. No loss of correction is observed, and a solid fusion is present despite wire failure.

Fig. 5-11B.

Forty-one patients underwent a single-stage procedure, and three patients, all adults, underwent multiple-stage procedures for rigid deformities.

Single-stage procedures were carried out in 28 adolescents with 32 curves. The average preoperative curve was 49.1 degrees, with an initial postoperative correction of 20.9 degrees. The final correction at follow-up was 22.8 degrees, with a loss of 1.7 degrees. The final correction was 53.5%. Average blood loss was 1629 ml in this group of adolescents using hypotensive anesthesia, and operative time averaged two hours and 45 minutes. There were no neurologic deficits, no infections, and no other serious complications in this group. At follow-up, no pseudarthroses have yet been detected. One patient sustained wire fatigue unilaterally, at the distal end vertebra. The fusion, however, was solid radiographically, and the patient was asymptomatic (Fig. 5-11).

Thirteen adult patients with 18 curves were managed with a single-stage procedure. Their preoperative curves averaged 47.3 degrees, with a range of 38 to 81 degrees. Initial postoperative correction averaged 30.7 degrees, with no loss of correction at follow-up. The percentage of correction was 35.1%. Estimated blood loss in this adult population was 2203 ml. Operative time averaged three-and-one-half hours.

Three adult patients with four curves underwent multistaged procedures for severe rigid deformities, which preoperatively averaged 96.5 degrees, ranging , from 70 to 134 degrees. Anterior release, Halo gravity traction, and posterior surgery were performed in two patients, and posterior and anterior osteotomies, culminating in posterior instrumentation and fusion, were carried out in one patient. The initial postoperative correction was 57.5 degrees, with no loss of correction at follow-up. The average correction was 49.4%.

Pseudarthroses occurred in two patients, both adults—one having a single-stage procedure, the other a two-stage procedure. Both underwent pseudarthrosis repair and revision of wires.

Instrument failures occurred in three patients, for an incidence of 18%; two sustained pseudarthroses and one went on to a solid fusion. In the adult group, there were no neurologic deficits, infections, or vascular complications. One patient with a severe rigid scoliosis of 135 degrees, who underwent a three-stage procedure, developed pneumonia with pleural effusion after the third stage, which prolonged her hospital stay.

All patients, both adolescents and adults, maintained physiologic sagittal curves. Postoperative immobilization was randomized to include partial immobilization in a custom fabricated TLSO, which was removed for bathing and sleeping, to no immobilization at all.

Comparison of Types of Postoperative Immobilization in Idiopathic Scoliosis

The first 27 patients who were surgically treated with segmental spinal instrumentation and posterior fusion were critically analyzed in an attempt to determine the effectiveness of the procedure and the necessity for postoperative immobilization. All patients underwent surgery without preoperative casting or traction.

Two groups were studied. Group One consisted of 15 patients who were immobilized six months postoperatively in a TLSO, which was removed for bathing and sleeping. Group Two consisted of 12 patients who were not immobilized. The average ages were 27 and 18 years, respectively. The follow-up was 11.3 months in Group One and 15.5 months in Group Two. The distribution of the curves and their preoperative measurements are demonstrated in Table 5-4. Postoperatively, initial correction was measured on the first standing radiograph, and final correction and percentage of correction on the latest follow-up standing radiograph. The values associated with both Group One and Group Two are seen in Table 5-5. The difference in the final percentage of correction is best, but not totally, explained by the fact that most of the nonimmobilized Group Two patients were operated on in the early part of the study, when spinal cord monitoring was not available. Sagittal curves were analyzed in both groups and found to be fairly similar (Table 5-6). Sagittal curves were maintained in the physiologic range and in the thoracic spine were improved.

TABLE 5-5

Comparison of Immobilization in Idiopathic Scoliosis

Curve	Initial Correction	Final Correction	% Correction
Group I			
T	30.3°	29.8°	49%
TL	27°	32°	47%
L	17.5°	18°	62%
D	34°/22.8°	33.8°/23.2°	40%/52%
Group II			
T	34.2°	33.4°	39%
TL	19°	23°	42%
L	17°	19°	52%
D	26.3°/26°	30.3°/31.3°	46%/39%

TABLE 5-6

Comparison of Immobilization in Idiopathic Scoliosis

	Preoperative	Initial	Final
Group I			
Kyphosis	24°	28°	33°
Lordosis	39°	35°	35°
Group II			
Kyphosis	25°	36°	36°
Lordosis	32°	33°	33°

The average loss of correction was analyzed according to two parameters. It was considered significant if more than three degrees were lost between initial and final follow-up films. First the entire study group was considered. Sixteen patients with 18 curves underwent instrumentation with 3/16-inch rods and had an average loss of correction of 2.5 degrees. Eleven patients with 17 curves were treated with one-quarter inch rods, with an average loss of correction of 2.3 degrees. Furthermore, there was little difference in the average final percentage of correction with either size rod (Table 5-7).

Secondly, loss of correction was analyzed according to whether the patients were immobilized postoperatively. One patient in Group One with a thoracolumbar

TABLE 5-7

Comparison of Immobilization in Idiopathic Scoliosis

	Ave % Correction
³⁄₁₆″ Rods	
16 patients	
18 curves	
47% correction	
¼″ Rods	
11 patients	
17 curves	
42.2% correction	

curve lost five degrees. At follow-up, this curve was solidly fused, and the patient did not experience instrument failure. In Group Two, loss of correction occurred in four patients without pseudarthroses. Four patients had distal wire failure: two with resultant pseudarthroses and two with resultant solid fusions seen on radiographic examination. Other than the above-mentioned instrument complications, there were no neurologic sequelae or infections in either group.

From the analysis of this small group of patients, certain preliminary conclusions can be drawn. First, there does not appear to be any significant difference in either the correction obtained or the loss of correction whether quarter-inch or ³⁄₁₆-inch rods are applied. Three of the distal wire failures in the nonimmobilized group occurred with one-quarter inch rods, however. It is postulated that perhaps increased stiffness of the quarter-inch rods produces a stress riser at the distal segment. Another possibility is that the 16-gauge double wires were overtightened and weakened at the junction of the twist and the loop.

Secondly, it is our belief that active patients with idiopathic scoliosis should be partially immobilized to prevent loss of correction and wire failure, which is more prone to develop in the nonimmobilized lumbar spine and which may lead to pseudarthrosis.

Thirdly, partial immobilization is more readily accepted by all patients, is more pleasing cosmetically, and allows improved personal hygiene; patients' activity and lifestyle are thus much less restricted.

In summary, segmental spinal instrumentation with Luque rods satisfactorily corrects idiopathic scoliosis when compared to Harrington rods and, more important, restores and preserves physiologic sagittal curves.

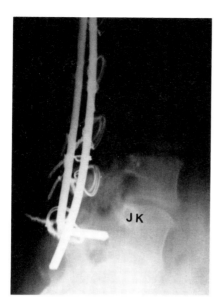

Fig. 5-12. J.K., a 43-year-old female with idiopathic scoliosis. Lateral tomograms nine months postoperatively demonstrate migration of the distal end of the rod, with an osseous reaction secondary to rod impingement on the sacral lamina. Although not well shown, wires were fatigued at L4 and L5 with resultant pseudarthroses. Reexploration and rod revision were necessary, with repair of failed fusion.

Disadvantages

What are the disadvantages of segmental spinal instrumentation? The most obvious and most formidable disadvantage of this technique is the necessity of wire placement within the spinal canal. Careful and meticulous operative technique and spinal cord monitoring with evoked potentials will certainly avoid serious neurologic complications. Long-range effects, however, pose another problem. If pseudarthroses occur, the absence of stress risers in the smooth L-rods will transfer stresses to either bone or wire, with resultant fracture or metal fatigue. This may lead to impingement of neural structures and possible damage. The fail-safe mechanism of hook dislodgement away from neural structures built into the Harrington system is not present when sublaminar wires are used. To date, neurologic signs and symptoms accompanying wire breakage have not occurred in this author's experience.

Another disadvantage of the double L-rod segmental system is the situation at distal end. Of necessity, a segment of rod must protrude over the distal and proximal L portions. This allows secure fixation of both rods to the lamina. In several instances, with the passage of time, settling of the instrumentation device has occurred, with elongation of the protruding ends and subsequent shortening of the construct. This is most likely due to soft tissue and bony erosion at the wire

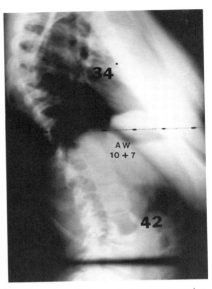

Fig. 5-13*A*. A.W., a 10-plus 7-year-old female with severe progressive 68° right thoracic idiopathic scoliosis.

B, Normal sagittal curves on x-ray examination.

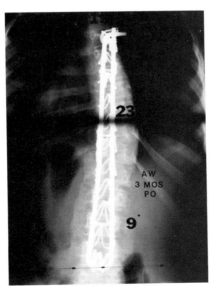

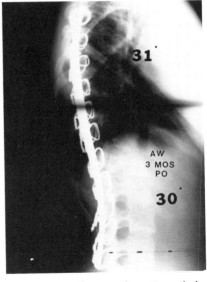

C, Correction with box-rod configuration three months postoperatively showing early spinal fusion taking place and a "cleaner" implant end distally.

D, Lateral x-ray three months postoperatively. Sagittal contours are well maintained with smooth transition distally between instrumented and uninstrumented vertebra.

sites. In the close quarters present in the lower lumbar spine, the remaining mobile segments can abut against the rod end and cause symptoms. Furthermore, if fusion to L5 is necessary, a protruding rod end may erode through the thin sacral lamina (Fig. 5-12). This problem can be corrected by a "cleaner" distal configuration in the Luque system. To this end, box configurations have been developed which may, in the long run, obviate this bothersome complication (Fig. 5-13). However, if settling, of necessity, takes place in the time required for spinal fusion, the stresses may be transferred to the distal wires, causing fatigue, or to the proximal segment where upward migration might take place. These are unanswered questions, since this newer construct is only in its initial phase of application.

Another theoretical disadvantage of the Luque system is that less bone stock is available for posterior fusion, when compared with the Harrington technique. Furthermore, greater amounts of bone graft are necessary to cover the transverse processes in sufficient quantity, especially in the lumbar spine. We do not feel that this is a disadvantage if meticulous facet fusion is performed, coupled with meticulous decortication. Our resultant fusions have hypertrophied and have appeared more than adequate on radiologic examination.

There is no question that operating time is increased because of the more demanding and exacting technique. Because of the increased time involved, blood loss is also increased. This theoretically poses a greater risk to the patient. In our series of 44 patients with idiopathic scoliosis, however, we have not found this to be the case. The added benefits of rigid internal fixation, allowing greater freedom and safety of nursing care and early mobilization, especially in the adult idiopathic population and the neuromuscular group, have negated the high rate of postoperative complications reported by others.

Summary

Spinal deformity surgery is one of the great challenges in Orthopedics. Once a stepchild, forgotten and avoided by most, it was adopted and renewed with vigor when Paul Harrington introduced his pioneering instrumentation, successfully and for the first time, in 1960.[29,30] It marked a milestone in scoliosis surgery, allowing walking in a Milwaukee brace or plaster cast soon after spinal fusion. Dr. Harrington developed his technique out of the need to help children who, afflicted with polio, developed severe spinal deformities. Despite inauspicious beginnings, it became the mainstay in the surgical management of scoliosis, through the recognition that meticulous fusion and casting technique are obligatory for its success. Eduardo Luque of Mexico City, in the early 1970s, found the need in his social environment to develop an instrumentation system that provided such rigid internal fixation that it permitted his patients to remain without postoperative immobilization while their spinal fusions healed. His trials and errors are the essence of this volume.

Each contributor to this volume has embraced this innovation—some more reservedly than others—and has taken it steps further in its continuing evolution, both in the laboratory and clinically. Careful scrutiny by these authors makes evident the many unknowns still to be solved. We are reminded that meticulous attention to detail is an absolute necessity in patient selection, curve compensation, fusion technique, and most important, the prevention of neurologic damage. Segmental spinal instrumentation is a technically demanding exercise. It should not be attempted by the uninitiated.

The concept of rigid segmental instrumentation is sound and proven. Segmental spinal instrumentation will undoubtedly become a basic in the armamentarium of the spinal surgeon. With time and basic investigation, Eduardo Luque's necessity may become a means for our patients' greater comfort and convenience.

Editor's Note

SSI as a method of rigid internal fixation is directly related to pathology, size of the individual patient, amount of correction obtained, quality of the bone, and length of the instrumentation. If arthrodesis is being used, there will always be a race between instrument failure and development of bony arthrodesis. The activity of the patient postoperatively, the size of the patient, the size of the rod used, and the amount of force applied to correct the deformity should all be taken into consideration in determining whether a patient should use external immobilization in the postoperative period. Again, individualization requires good judgment.

One of the important limitations of this type of spine surgery is adequate hospital facilities. The possibility of danger is increased when a complete work-up of the patient is not done. It is my experience that not only must the surgeon have experience and manual dexterity, but he also must be able to command complete attention from his entire surgical team throughout the entire intervention.

Preoperative distraction has not been useful in our hands. Nevertheless, halo wheelchair distraction after anterior release and before posterior instrumentation has definite validity, especially in elongating the soft tissues.

Reference is made by Dr. Taddonio to the deformity of the posterior elements in kyphosis. It must be emphasized that due to this elongation of the posterior column, shortening procedures are used to avoid elongation of the neural canal on correction (Fig. 5-14). In an ideal model with balanced correction and correct immobilization, most of the osseous graft should lay where it is under the least strain. This would probably be the concave side of the three-dimensional deformity (Figs. 5-15 and 5-16).

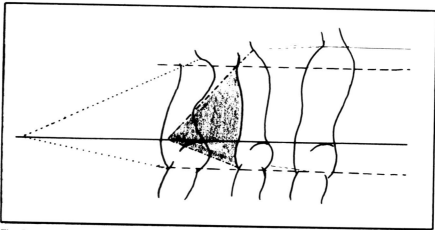

Fig. 5-14A. In the normal standing posture in the sagittal plane, the trunk outline is made by the spinal column behind and the anterior abdominal wall and cartilagenous and osseous thoracic components. In a normal individual the angle between the T1-T2 interspace and the lop of the manubrium is ± 15°, figure far right. In a patient with spine deformity this angle is increased by the posterior kyphos. Figure far left. In a patient who has been corrected by elongating the spinal column this angle is even more increased due to the fixed length of the anterior structures. This provokes a "sucking in" of the semimobile lateral and anterior structures as they try to adjust to the uneven stretch, central figure.

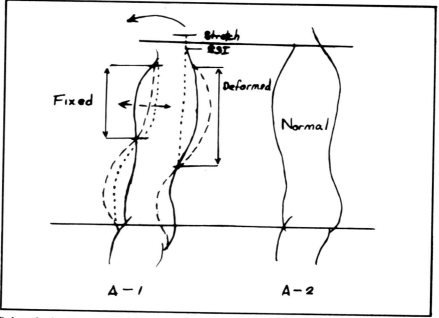

B, Lengthening the spine to obtain correction will suck in the anterior structures (sternum and ribs), since they have a fixed length. Shortening procedures are important to give a balanced, normal sagittal alignment.

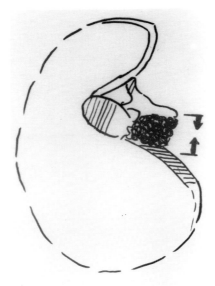

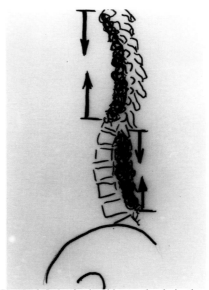

Fig. 5-15. The ideal position of an osseous graft is on the concave side of the remaining deformity. Considering the 3D deformity in scoliosis, this usually means on the concave side of the curve. With a kyphotic component, however, it would be on the convex anterior aspect of the vertebral body.

Fig. 5-16. In kyphosis without arthrodesis, the compression site is anterior to the neural canal; in lordosis, it is posterior to the neural elements.

Each one of the authors has developed a special technique for passing and fixing wires safely on the laminas. My own preference is to use closed-loop 18-gauge wire passed under the lamina and threaded through itself. This avoids all possibility of damage to the cord in the process of manipulation. Once the arthrodesis is done, the bead is cut off at each level. The rod is introduced between the wires, which are in turn twisted over the rod, thus locking the entire system. We do our arthrodesis before passing the wires.

Instrumentation is no substitute for a good fusion technique. In using double wires, Dove has shown that their strength is similar to that of wires of thicker gauge; eg, double 18-gauge wires are as resistant as a single 16-gauge wire. It must be emphasized, though, that to tighten both double wires evenly, a hook twister with distraction must be used. If done with any other type of clamp, the twist will result in a one-wire work situation.

The wire-bone interface is of extreme importance, especially in children and osteoporotic bone. Looping the lamina eliminates problems at the wire-bone contact point. As far as wire fixation on the sacrum, the S1 facet seems to be the strongest bony substance, and a wire hold should always be placed there. If possible, a hold should also be used at the S1-L5 level or at S1-S2.

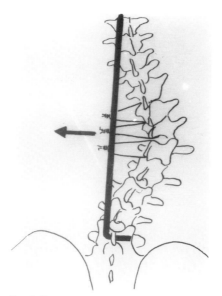

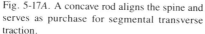

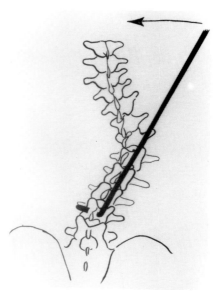

Fig. 5-17*A*. A concave rod aligns the spine and serves as purchase for segmental transverse traction.

B, A convex bar produces pressure at the apex and brings the flexible ends of the curve to the bar.

It is important to note that in obtaining correction, the concave rod aligns the deformity, while the convex bar has the greatest corrective force. This is accomplished by putting pressure on the apex of the deformity and bringing the flexible ends to the rod (Fig. 5-17). We wish to make the most of our correction with a broad rod-to-bone contact, not by wire pulling. Correspondingly, most of the correction at the apex should be done by the convex rod, while the alignment of the flexible end should be done by the concave rod. The end wires on the convex rod and the apical wires on the concave rod will ultimately break if not adequately treated. To avoid undue stress on the wire, distraction should be used at a 45° angle, and the wire twist should end directly over the rod.

Box-type rods have been used in the lower back since 1976. They have been used for scoliosis and fractures since 1979. Their application is more technically demanding, but as we obtain more skill and better tools, they will probably be used more often. It is interesting to note that in every series, rods that have been inserted under stress keep working but will eventually fatigue, even in the presence of a solid arthrodesis (Fig. 5-18).

Dr. Taddonio's scientific analysis of his case material shows the need for anterior surgery and shortening procedures. It seemed obvious to all of us in 1977 that SSI was a tremendously corrective force in two planes, the AP and the sagittal. We all expected correction in the axial plane. We also had illusions that by creating balanced three-dimensional correction and making compensatory curves, anterior surgery would be avoided. It is obvious that we are all still learning and are far from

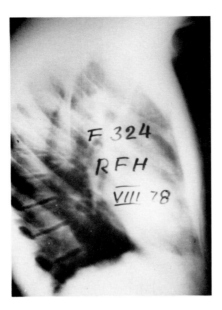

Fig. 5-18A. A 29-year-old male with a round back.

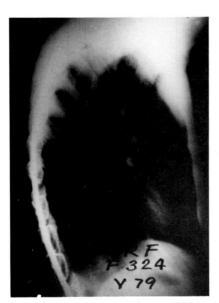

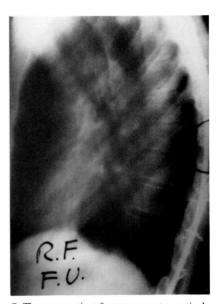

B, Postoperative correction nine months later after SSI and Hibbs-Risser arthrodesis. Notice how on elongation of the spinal column (correction without shortening procedures), the anterior chest wall is retreated inward.

C, The same patient four years postoperatively with a solid posterior arthrodesis. There is no loss of correction, but there is a fractured bar due to fatigue.

having all the answers. Personally, I find myself doing more anterior surgery (corpectomies and diskectomies), more posterior surgery at the apex of the curves, and more alignment in all planes.

In our personal experience, apical rotation has not been affected, even with extensive anterior-posterior releases. We have changed the thoracic image, however, by transposition of the spine, concave rib osteotomies, and convex transverse release. The use of postoperative arthrosis is relative to each patient, each disorder, and the geography of each medical center.

References

1. Luque ER: The anatomic basis and development of segmental spinal instrumentation. Spine 7:256-259, 1982.

2. Allen BL, Ferguson RL: The Galveston technique for L rod instrumentation of the scoliotic spine. Spine 7:276-284, 1982.

3. Taddonio RF: Segmental spinal instrumentation in the management of neuromuscular spinal deformity. Spine 7:305-311, 1982.

4. Sullivan JA, Conner SB: Comparison of Harrington instrumentation and segmental spinal instrumentation in the management of neuromuscular spinal deformity. Spine 7:299-304, 1982.

5. Herring JA, Wenger DR: Segmental spinal instrumentation. A preliminary report of 40 consecutive cases. Spine 7:285-298, 1982.

6. Luque ER, Cassis N, Ramirez-Wiella G: Segmental spinal instrumentation in the treatment of fracture of the thoraco lumbar spine. Spine 7:312-317, 1982.

7. Luque ER: Segmental spinal instrumentation for correction of scoliosis. Clinical Orthopaedics 163:192-198, 1982.

8. Bonnett C, Brown JC, Grow T: Thoracolumbar scoliosis in cerebral palsy. J Bone Jt Surg 58A:328-336, 1976.

9. Bonnett C, Brown JC, Perry J, et al: Evolution of treatment of paralytic scoliosis at Rancho Los Amigos Hospital. J Bone Jt Surg 57A:206-215, 1975.

10. Blamer GA, MacEwen GD: The incidence and treatment of scoliosis and cerebral palsy. J Bone Jt Surg 52B:134-137, 1970.

11. Harrington PR: The management of scoliosis by spine instrumentation. South Med J 31:367-376, 1963.

12. Harrington PR: The spine in the handicapped child. Am J Ortho 6:156-164, 1964.

13. Wenger DR, Carollo JJ, Wilkerson JA: Biomechanics of scoliosis correction by segmental spinal instrumentation. Spine 7:260-264, 1982.

14. Wenger DR, Carollo JJ, Wilkerson JA, et al: Laboratory testing of segmental instrumentation versus traditional Harrington instrumentation for scoliosis treatment. Spine 7:265-269, 1982.

15. Taddonio RF, Weller K, Appel M: A comparison of patients managed with and without postoperative immobilization following segmental spinal instrumentation with Luque rods: A preliminary report. Presented at the 18th Annual Meeting of the Scoliosis Research Society, New Orleans, Louisiana, September 1983.

16. Luque ER: The correction of postural curves of the spine. Spine 7:270-275, 1982.

17. Moe JH, Denis F: The iatrogenic loss of lumbar lordosis. Ortho Trans 1:2, 1977.

18. Goldstein L, Ginsberg H, Haake WV: Back pain in postoperative idiopathic scoliosis—long term follow-up. Ortho Trans 2:2, 1978.

19. Taddonio RF, Sternberg R, Schultz RJ: Preoperative evaluation of the patient with spinal deformity using Swan-Ganz catheterization. Ortho Trans 7:1, 1983.

20. Moe JH: Methods of correction and surgical technique in scoliosis. Ortho Clin N Am 2:17, 1972.

21. Allen BL: Personal communication, 1981.

22. Bradford DS: The surgical management of patients with Scheuermann's disease: A review of twenty-four cases managed by combined anterior and posterior spine fusion. J Bone Jt Surg 62A:705-712, 1980.

23. Winter RB, Lovell WW, Moe JH: Excessive thoracic lordosis and loss of pulmonary function in patients with idiopathic scoliosis. J Bone Jt Surg 57A:972-977, 1975.

24. Leider LL, Moe JH, Winter RB: Early ambulation after the surgical treatment of idiopathic scoliosis. J Bone Jt Surg 55A:1003-1015, 1973.

25. Mir SR, Cole JR, Lardone J, et al: Early ambulation following spinal fusion and Harrington instrumentation in idiopathic scoliosis. Clin Ortho 110:54-62, 1975.

26. Erwin WD, Dickson JH, Harrington PR: The postoperative management of scoliosis patients treated with Harrington instrumentation and fusion. J Bone Jt Surg 58A:479-482, 1976.

27. Ponder RC, Dickson JH, Harrington PR, et al: Results of Harrington instrumentation and fusion in the adult idiopathic scoliosis patient. J Bone Jt Surg 57A:797-801, 1975.

28. Swank S, Lonstein JE, Moe JH, et al: Surgical treatment of adult scoliosis—A review of two hundred and twenty-two cases. J Bone Jt Surg 63A:268-287, 1981.

29. Harrington PR: Surgical instrumentation for management of scoliosis. J Bone Jt Surg 42A:1448, 1960.

30. Harrington PR: Correction and internal fixation by spine instrumentation. J Bone Jt Surg 44A:591-610, 1962.

Paralytic Scoliosis

6

Classification

There are three types of paralytic scoliosis: neuromuscular, myopathic, and congenital.

1. *Neuromuscular or Neuropathic* has the following subtypes.
   a. Low motor neuron lesion, as in poliomyelitis.
   b. High motor neuron lesion, as in cerebral palsy.
   c. Other (syringomyelia).

2. *Myopathic* scoliosis can be divided into four types.
   a. Progressive, as in muscular dystrophy.
   b. Static, as in amyotonia.
   c. Others, such as Friedreich's ataxia.
   d. Unilateral amelia.

3. *Congenital* scoliosis is due to spinal vertebra and cord deformity caused by abnormal development.

Scoliosis, Kyphosis and Lordosis Caused by Myelodysplasia

The effect that these diseases have on the spine is very serious, owing to the fact that their onset is at a very early age. They will, therefore, cause deformities in the thorax and in the tone of the diaphragm, as well as affecting the stability required for sitting, standing, or walking. These disorders lead to respiratory and cardiac disturbances, which ultimately cause the patient's death.[2,3,8,10,16,23,26] Sometimes truly dramatic situations occur, such as progressive muscular dystrophy, in which the patient is unable to remain seated owing to spinal pain yet is unable to lie down owing to severe respiratory distress.

In disorders involving paralysis of the legs and hips, and in some disorders involving sensitivity, nonsurgical treatment is even more difficult. Either the use of practically any type of cast is impossible, or extremely costly braces of little practical use are required, such as wheelchairs with molded backs.

We must bear in mind that some of these disorders, such as sequelae of poliomyelitis, are still prevalent in countries with little in the way of economic, social, and cultural resources, where it is very difficult to obtain medical care and attention. Therefore, definitive treatment in a single hospitalization is required. Each patient requires different treatment in accordance with his general condition, and objectives must be carefully planned so as not to undertreat him or to provide impractical and useless overtreatment. Questions such as the following should be asked: Can the patient walk? Can he sit? Does he walk with crutches? With braces? Will he remain confined to a wheelchair? Does he have sufficient intellectual capacity? How much independence can the patient be given? There is no one answer to these questions; neither is there one means of treatment. Yet the stability of the spine is the first step in treatment in each of these cases.

Evaluation of the Paralytic Scoliosis Patient

All patients suffering from paralysis must undergo an exhaustive muscular evaluation. This is the basis for planning the treatment prior to spinal stabilization, as well as for determining the extent of spinal fixation. An analysis of lung function is necessary in order to determine the surgical risks and diagnosis. It may be safely said that all paralytic scoliosis patients suffer from poor respiratory function, independent of the location of the principal curve.

Psychologic examination, IQ testing, evaluation of motivation, and socioeconomic studies are performed next. The x-ray evaluation of the deformity is done with the patient standing, seated supine, and bending right or left, and flexion or extension films are obtained in cases of pelvic obliquity or abnormal kyphosis or lordosis. With the foregoing, we chart a course of treatment, including correction

Table 6-1.

General Principals of Scoliosis as a Poliomyelitis Sequela

Dorsal lumbar curves, including the pelvis, occurred in 57.7% of 359 paralytic scoliosis cases. Lumbar curves, including the pelvis, numbered 23.4%, and dorsal curves numbered 14.5%. The first two percentages together totaled 81.1%, which explains the fixation of the pelvis in the majority of patients.

The shortening of the pelvic extremities occurs in 75% of the cases. No direct relationship was found between the shortening and the side of the curve.

The average degree of scoliosis is 78.8° and varies between 15° and 150°. In 96.26%, the disease starts when the child is six months to three years old, although in severe cases the disease might start when the child is one month old or when he is seven years old. The range of occurrence in both sexes is 1 to 1. (Mexico City Shriners' Hospital, 1962-1974.)

---

of contractures, application of traction, and the use of casts against the curves with wedges to correct them. Surgery will provide a greater degree of spinal correction before segmental spinal instrumentation (SSI) is begun.

In formulating a program of respiratory exercises in accordance with the etiology and the patient's age, it must be remembered that vital capacity decreases with the use of casts, while the use of cephalic traction in the seated position (halo-chair) or halo-femoral traction improves respiratory conditions.[23,25]

For the paralytic patient, nonsurgical spine treatment may be more aggressive than simply early fixation and correction, depending on the etiology, spinal curve flexibility, and cardiopulmonary condition.

Dependent SSI

Poliomyelitis Sequelae

For patients who suffer from imbalance and absence of muscular support, the use of plastic or plaster corsets or the use of the Milwaukee brace for a prolonged period of time is useless. Alterations in pulmonary physiology and a decrease in the ability to walk or to remain seated would result, and in general terms a decline in lifestyle would be observed.

The goal to meet should be the improvement of the patient. In order to reach this, it is necessary to take care of each patient's problems individually, to apply the suitable treatment for each case, and to balance the spinal curves. During the last ten years, the use of SSI has been a satisfactory help in giving balance to the spine, and in nearly all cases the use of external supports becomes unnecessary. This also increases the respiratory function and brings an immediate improvement in the patient's life.

Length of Fixation

The length of fixation is determined according to the scoliotic curves, the presence of abnormal kyphosis or lordosis, and muscular conditions. The proximal region generally has the best musculature and better spinal support (Fig. 6-1). One manner of finding the area to be measured radiologically is to locate the proximal spinal vertebra parallel to the floor and neutral, which usually indicates a normal zone. The fixation should be long enough to sustain the correction of the kyphotic or lordotic deformity. From the clinical standpoint, the spine is stable when the musculature is properly balanced and sustains the column. Muscular evaluation is therefore very important. We require several parameters for evaluation of the length of fixation. It must be based on the musculature, principally the scapular belt, and three-dimensional x-rays. One should especially watch for scoliosis, kyphosis, rotation, trunk stability, and head-to-pelvis alignment and balance. Except in growing children, articular facet resection and laminar decortication should be performed, along with autologous grafts wherever possible.

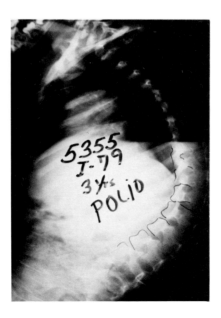

Fig. 6-1A to D. Female patient, age three, affected in all four extremities and the trunk. She has scoliosis (80° Cobb) from the cervical spine to the sacrum, kyphosis of 80° from the cervical spine to the sacrum, a history of respiratory ailments and pneumonia every two to four weeks, and a poor general condition. Following correction with SSI (C and D), the patient can sit without discomfort and is dramatically free of respiratory symptoms two years after surgical treatment.

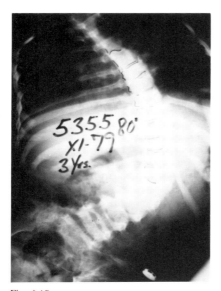

Fig. 6-1*B*.

Fig. 6-1*C*.

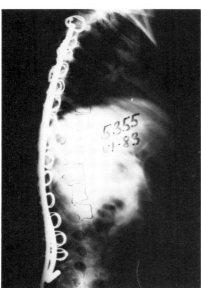

Fig. 6-1*D*.

If the curve is rigid or excessively severe and is 50% corrected with a severe residual curve remaining, spine-shortening surgery is desirable. Resection of intervertebral disks or resection of one or more vertebrae will increase spinal mobility and the degree of correction. Leaving a curve of 60° or more is of little practical value following such extensive and high-risk surgery.

Pelvic obliquity should always be corrected. Contractures should be removed, and a fascia lata tensor section in the hip should be performed. The iliopsoas and articular joint of the hip as well as the lumbar muscle should also be sectioned. A Calot cast should be left in place for two weeks prior to fixing the spine, thus making possible a greater degree of correction. Rigid pelvic obliquities may require a resection of the fifth lumbar vertebra. For our purpose, use of halo-femoral traction is *limited to cases of respiratory restriction,* and we consider use of halo-cephalic/halo-pelvic traction to be of little value. Highly practical is halo-chair or halo-ambulatory (Stagnara) traction.

Reports of correction using the Dwyer procedure imply reducing spinal length in resecting intervertebral disks. The same effect may be achieved by resecting one or more vertebrae without Dwyer instrumentation, reducing the time of surgery and the risks.

The stability of the trunk, the head-pelvis alignment (with shoulders parallel to the pelvis), and balanced curves in the three dimensions (scoliosis, kyphosis, lordosis, rotation) will have a positive effect on the patient's physical, psychologic, and social well-being.

For growing patients who require surgery, consideration must be given to the possibility of subsequent reoperations. In the case of highly flexible curves that are less than 20° after correction, a straight single subperiosteal convex-sided rod will be used, without dissection on the concave side. If the residual curve is 20° to 30°, the use of a concave rod will provide greater apex traction and may improve correction. If the residual curves are greater than 30°, the use of the concave-convex double rod is best. In addition, if pelvic fixation is required, two L-shaped rods are necessary,

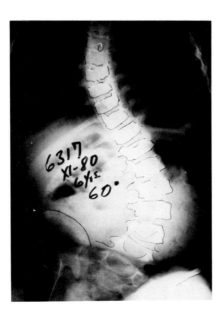

Fig. 6-2A to E. Male patient, age six, with pelvic obliquity and thoracolumbar kyphosis. He walks with difficulty using pelvic braces and crutches. The spine is fixed without arthrodesis, correcting the pelvic obliquity and creating lordosis. With this, his walking improved notably, becoming easier, and he can walk short distances without crutches. With no loss of correction, growth of the spine is possible in the area near the rods.

There is an error here, however—short fixation. Three additional vertebrae should have been included (Shriners Hospital, Mexico City Unit, Case No. 3617).

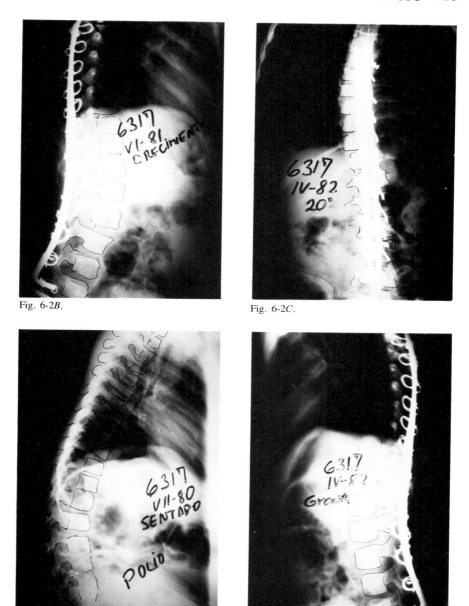

Fig. 6-2*B*.

Fig. 6-2*C*.

Fig. 6-2*E*.

Fig. 6-2*F*.

since a single L-shaped rod does not provide sufficient fixation. Spinal fixation without arthrodesis in growing patients permits continued growth (with sliding of the rods) (Fig. 6-2).[7,17,19,21,29]

Postoperative Treatment

Postoperative treatment is individual in nature, in accordance with the type of curve and fixation obtained. In growing patients with a residual curve of less than 30°, sitting, standing, walking, or any combination is possible if their muscular condition permits. We have used Risser-type antigravity casts on those patients who have already undergone extensive surgery to correct a previous procedure or have an enucleation of vertebral bodies with rigid curves. Corrections of 50% to 90% have been obtained. All these patients were ambulatory. If the patient remains in bed for a longer period of time, this will help him recover from a Soutter, Yount, or other procedure. The fact that the patient is in bed will diminish stress on a recently operated spine; this can be used to advantage if procedures requiring longer bed rest are planned. The use of antibiotics both during and after surgery reduces the possibility of infection and whenever possible they should be used for ten days following surgery (Fig. 6-3).

Complications

The possibility of infection should be no greater than .25%. Other possibilities, such as dura mater lesion, excessive bleeding, and transitory cutaneous hyperesthesias, will occur at a rate of less than 1.5%. Transitory cutaneous hyperesthesias are due to radicular traction; in correcting angulation and rotation, they appear principally in the lumbar region.[7,15,17-20,22,25,29] Vascular obstruction of the duodenum may occur due to correction of lumbar kyphosis. Severe corrective lordosis is a possibility in very thin patients and, if not given timely and adequate treatment, may cause death.

The possibility of neurologic complications may arise in those patients requiring exclusively instrumentation-based correction with a shortening procedure. We have proposed correction of not more than 10% of contrary stress as seen on dynamic x-rays. Other methods of correction are used a priori, including SSI exclusively, as a means of rigid internal fixation. Another possibility is that a technical error may occur in introducing the rods at the sacral level (due to a decrease in anterior-posterior diameter and the convex shape of the sacrum). For these purposes, we recommend that a complete view be obtained. A transverse perforation should be made in the sacrum instead of two holes, which limit the view of the sacral roots. In this way, there would be no risk of entangling the roots and the wire.

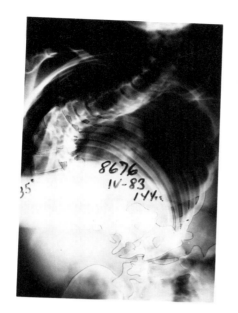

Fig. 6-3*A* to *E*. Female patient, age 16. Scoliosis of 135° and rigid thoracolumbar kyphosis of 115° are present (*A* and *B*). Resection of the vertebral body of T11 and T9 was done by an anterior approach (*C*). The patient proved able to shed her cast after four months (*D* and *E*). This patient used a Risser-type cast for four months (Shriners Hospital, Mexico City Unit, Case No. 8676).

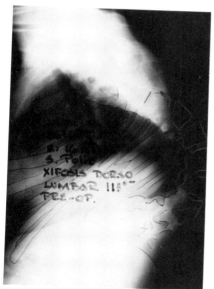

Fig. 6-3*B*.

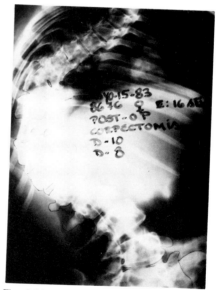

Fig. 6-3*C*.

The risk of pseudarthrosis must be no greater than 10%. This condition must be considered a syndrome that includes rupture of the material, loss of correction, and pain. In our experience, up to 21% of rods have broken with neither loss of correction nor subjective discomfort of any kind, with no need for new surgery

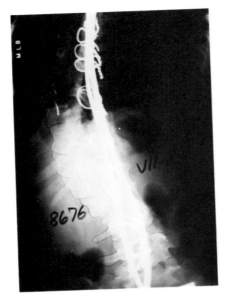

Fig. 6-3D.

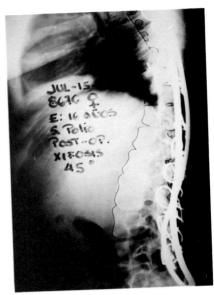

Fig. 6-3E.

Fig. 6-4A to D. Female patient, age 15, with 97° scoliosis. Good correction was obtained, but nine months later the rod broke on the convex side at the distal angle, with neither pain nor loss of correction. A solid arthrodesis was done three years later. It was an error to use straight rods, with no kyphosis or lordosis. This was not considered pseudarthrosis.

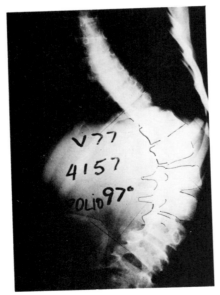

Fig. 6-4A.

after several years of follow-up. In view of this, we have not considered this pseudarthrosis. The L rod sustaining pelvic obliquity has broken in two cases, with no loss of correction or symptoms.

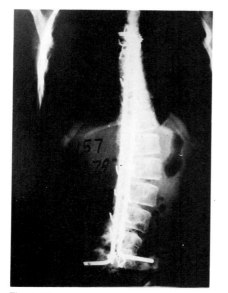

Fig. 6-4*B*.

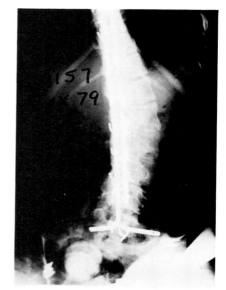

Fig. 6-4*C*.

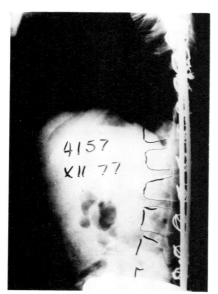

Fig. 6-4*D*.

It is probable that this breakage of material is due to fatigue caused by the continuous union of opposing forces held together with the belts joining both bars, rather than being the result of organic pressures. We must accept that the spine continues growing at the same time that the fusion is taking place, causing a greater stress than the one present while the fixation and maintenance of the correction occur (Fig. 6-4).

We have, unfortunately, read in the literature reports of poor results with Harrington rods and wires while the technique was being developed. We must therefore emphasize *the maintenance of both physiologic curves and the balance of residual curves,* which reduce the stress on the material, decreasing the risk of pseudarthrosis. We must avoid combining the defects of the two techniques: straight bars and distraction in two points, where the hooks become dislocated due to the lateral pressure. The two opposite forces, traction and flexion, cancel each other.

Results

The degree of correction varies in accordance with the methods used to achieve such correction, with the average being 65%. Eighty-nine and nine-tenths percent of the patients are ambulatory using either crutches or braces. When the correction was highly important, Risser antigravity casts were used in 14% of the cases. Patients who were nonambulatory owing to severe postparalytic complications numbered 10.1%. Pseudarthrosis occurred in 7%, and second reoperations for pseudarthrosis averaged 3%.

Average bleeding: The average amount of bleeding is 1200 cc.

Average time of surgery: Operating on ten vertebrae normally takes approximately 3.10 hours.

Conclusions

With the use of SSI, the occurrence of pseudarthrosis and general morbidity have diminished considerably, permitting early walking. Both respiratory and overall physical rehabilitation start immediately. The increase in vital capacity is due to the maintenance of normal kyphotic and lordotic curves. This permits a normal diaphragmatic range of motion, since it maintains its tone even when affected by the original disorder.

The principal indication is to provide a rigid internal fixation system to avoid the necessity for long periods of bed rest or the use of external supports. A decrease in the risk of pseudarthrosis is also an advantage. This has been achieved with this technique without increasing either morbidity or mortality vis-à-vis other techniques.

SSI achieves the following objectives:

1. Attains rigid fixation that can be used with or without arthrosis.

2. Has the versatility to mold the bars in three dimensions, allowing a better in toto balance.

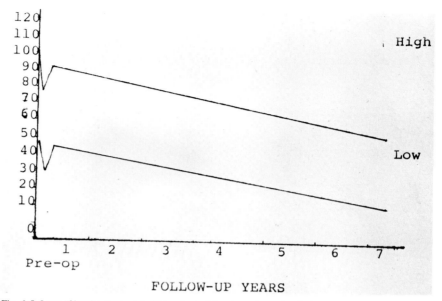

Fig. 6-5. Loss of lumbar lordosis in 114 patients following spine arthrodesis, with seven years of follow-up. Vital capacity as measured with the Collins Vitalometer was average in seated, standing, and recumbent positions.

3.   Directs spine growth toward a physiologic position in growing patients.

4.   In most cases, renders the use of external supports unnecessary.

5.   Improves the cardiorespiratory capacity.

6.   Combined with other procedures (spine shortening), can be used as a means of correction.

7.   Definitely improves life expectancy and the quality of life.

Observations

Vital Capacity

In the Mexico City unit of the Shriners' Hospital, various surgical techniques have been employed, including those of Albee, Hibbs-Risser, Harrington, and Luque. A study of the vital capacity of these patients has been conducted. A decline in postoperative vital capacity, which is both frequent and progressive, was found when lumbar lordosis was lost. This was a frequent occurrence from 1960 to

1970, before rod-molding had become a surgical reality (Fig. 6-5 and 6-6). The explanation for this is that the diaphragm is a dome-shaped muscle that loses its form with the disappearance of normal lumbar lordosis. This mechanical deformity decreases the diaphragm's range of motion in the thoracic cavity and therefore diminishes vital capacity. One of the most vital contributions of SSI is the maintenance of physiologic curves, which translates into a long-range improvement in vital capacity, as opposed to the progressive long-term decline seen when straight rods are used.[23,26,29]

Growing Patients

In growing patients younger than 11 years of age, production of lumbar lordosis has been observed even if straight rods were used. This is explained by the presence of physiologic growing zones, including the diaphragm.

Progressive Muscular Dystrophy and Spinal Deformities Associated with Hereditary Neurologic Conditions

This group of disorders takes on the form of either hereditary, progressive, and symmetric muscular paralysis caused by the degeneration of horn cells, or else a primary muscular disorder with similar clinical behavior and prognosis. The spinal curve or deformity pattern is highly variable in each of these cases. There is, however, a lumbar predomination (which includes the pelvis), in addition to scoliosis with lumbar or dorsal lordosis and lumbar kyphosis. In progressive muscular dystrophies, Wilkins and Gibson name five groups, of which the most stable, Group Five, is difficult to diagnose. In the face of imminent respiratory deficiency, this group is a likely prospect for surgical correction.

There are several names for spinal atrophy, such as Werdnig-Hoffmann disease, Kugelberg-Welander disease, or congenital amyotonia. Few cases survive beyond six years of age except with the Kugelberg-Welander form, which develops at a later age but generally brings about severe spinal deformities. With progressive muscular dystrophy (Duchenne type), the patient may be unable to remain seated owing to a severe spinal deformity and unable to recline because of respiratory distress. In every case, respiratory distress is the cause of death in these patients, leading to congestive right heart failure, retention of fluids, and pneumonia. The decision of whether to perform spinal surgery on these patients is based on the following considerations:

1.   The progression of spinal deformity. Spinal fixation greatly improves the quality

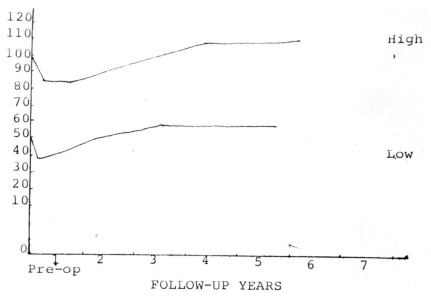

Fig. 6-6. Spine fixation caused lumbar lordosis in 95 patients, with five years of follow-up (Shriners Hospital, Mexico City Unit).

of the patient's life, allows him to sit, and improves his ventilatory capacity, independent of his age.

2. Progressive decline in vital capacity. This is also independent of the patient's age. Even in cases of moderate deformities, the spine must be fixed before surgery becomes impossible because of respiratory distress. We use as a guideline the decline from 50% to 40% of vital capacity under periodic quarterly observation. If a drop occurs, surgery is required.

3. Increases in dorsal lordosis, lumbar kyphosis, and pelvic obliquity and declines in vital capacity are always progressive and develop in parallel.

Length of Fixation

In the experience of the Mexico City Unit of the Shriners' Hospital and the Germán Díaz Lombardo Hospital, the fixation should be sufficient to keep the head, trunk, and pelvis stable according to the extent of the deformity, the ambulatory capacity, and the age. Clinical results of the fusion of the cervical column to the sacrum are highly encouraging; the quality of the patient's life improves noticeably, as confirmed by the patients themselves and their relatives. When we first started using SSI, the length of fusion was from T1 to S1, but we often found ourselves extending the fusion to C2 or C1. If the extension was up to C1, we would leave C1 unfused (Fig. 6-7).

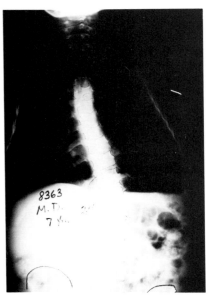 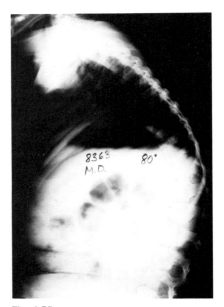

Fig. 6-7A and B. Male patient, age 7, with muscular dystrophy and spinal imbalance, 20° thoracolumbar scoliosis, and 80° kyphosis. Four months of postoperative treatment resulted in good balance in the physiologic curves and a stable pelvis. Fixation was performed from C3 to S4. The patient and his parents are very satisfied (C and D) (Shriners Hospital, Mexico City Unit, Case No. 8363).

Fig. 6-7B.

SSI is especially useful for several reasons:

1.   Rigid internal fixation, allowing the patient to sit in the immediate postoperative stage if respiratory disorders so require.

2.   Pelvic correction and stabilization not requiring use of external supports.

3.   Immediate initiation of ventilatory and general musculoskeletal rehabilitation.

4.   Avoidance of the use of molds or special braces in wheelchairs.

Conclusions

1.   Long fusions from C2 to S1 are not to be feared if one is maintaining the normal dorsal kyphosis and lumbar lordotic curves.

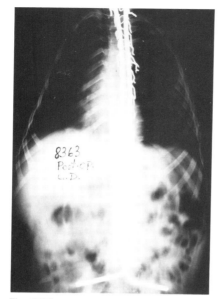

Fig. 6-7C.

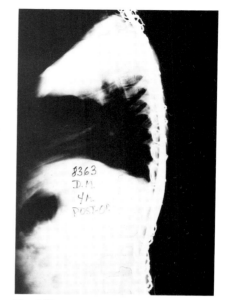

Fig. 6-7D.

2. Fixation at an early age is also not to be feared if it gives the patient a better quality of life and reduces the risk of surgery.

3. The fixation should be performed when the patient has ceased to be ambulatory, whenever possible.

4. The kyphotic-lordotic balance should be maintained in order to ensure proper trunk equilibrium while the patient is seated. Lumbar lordosis must be longer and more accentuated in order to maintain equilibrium in patients while standing.

5. Anterior-approach surgery is rarely indicated, while good corrections may be obtained using only the posterior approach.

Myelodysplasia

The most severe and most difficult to treat deformities are probably those caused by spina bifida and myelodysplasia. The high morbidity and mortality rates in these patients, who are frequently affected mentally, pose an ethical problem difficult to resolve.

The age of onset of these deformities is frequently so early that the decision to perform arthrodesis and the consequent shortening of the trunk involves many technical and ethical limitations. However, reports favoring early surgery and treatment are generally accepted, since the natural evolution of these deformities is well known.[13,24,28,30]

In the Mexico City Shriners' Hospital, spinal deformities occur in 58% of the cases of myelodysplasia. Before the patient reaches ten years of age, they are well established and foster the poor general condition of patients. Urinary tract infections occur in 97% of cases, pressure sores in 14%, and a decline in vital capacity of 20% to 60% in all patients. All these patients suffer from pelvic instability, and all require pelvic fixation in order to permit the use of braces or to assume the sitting position.

SSI offers, as additional advantages, the possibility of not using outside support, an increase in rigid internal immobility, and a decrease in the risk of pseudarthrosis. Technically, the difficulties in SSI are greater if there is deficiency in the posterior arches, longer surgical exposure of some trophic tissues, or skin defects.

Preoperative Treatment

Preoperative treatment should be focused on improving the patient's general condition, which in these patients is habitually poor; on treating such contaminating conditions as urinary tract infection; on treatment of pressure sores on the thoracic and pelvic members; and on plastic surgery.

Y incisions to prevent areas of cutaneous defects provide good access to posterolateral elements. Straight incisions may be made when the cutaneous defects do not cause deterioration in the epidermis and are not too severe. In order to hold the wires in place, we use neural foramina or the transverse process. The iliac crest fixation will be performed on the same side as that on which the rod is placed. A wire may be passed into the posterior and superior iliac crest in order to hold the L-shaped rod in place toward the sides, preventing medial displacement.

The length of fixation should be extended until sound elements, both muscularly and structurally stable, are located. This will correct such abnormal compensatory curves as dorsal hyperlordosis, will add homologous or autologous grafts, or both, sufficient for the requirements of each case in order to obtain an abundant bone bridge in the defective area, and will enable one to perform the fixation in normal, stable elements without fusion in order to lessen the possibilities of a resultant short thorax.

Prior to SSI, surgical methods using an anterior approach, such as "kypho" resection, intervertebral disk resection, common anterior ligament section, and Dwyer instrumentation, will be indicated. The surgeon must individualize them for each particular case. Posterior approach cord resection runs the grave risk of profuse hemorrhaging and death, and this is therefore proscribed.

Postoperative Treatment

Antibiotics must continue to be administered during the time required for the surgical wound to heal. Treatment of bladder disorders, adequate nursing care, frequent changes in posture, and the cleansing of anal incontinence decrease the possibilities of infecting the wound.

Early sitting and the use of braces by the patient are frequent possibilities with SSI, and there is no need for external supports, whether plastic casts, molds, or some other means. Walking or sitting within a week following surgery, or even earlier, is allowed.

Results

A direct consequence of SSI has been a rapid rehabilitation, varying from sitting in a wheelchair to enjoying greater independence in mobilization, dressing, and eating. The patient's general condition improves noticeably, and mentally there is a feeling of well-being and independence that might possibly have never before existed. This is also due in large measure to the fact that no external supports are used. The ambulatory patient may be equipped with braces for his pelvic area, and with the use of crutches, the load on the spine is decreased.

Follow-up time is short for this type of very young patient, whose average age is eight years. The short-term results are also encouraging.

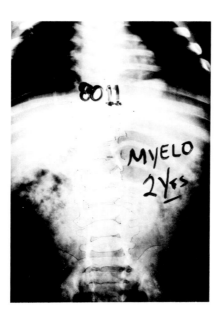

Fig. 6-8A to C. Male patient, age 2, with myelomeningocele from T11 to the sacrum. Rigid kyphosis is seen in evolution in D and E. Posterior-approach correction with posterior-approach resection of the vertex of the kyphosis and fixation were done at the same time. A plastic brace was used in the immediate postoperative treatment (Shriners Hospital, Mexico City Unit, Case No. 8011).

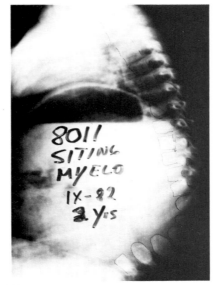

Fig. 6-8*B*.

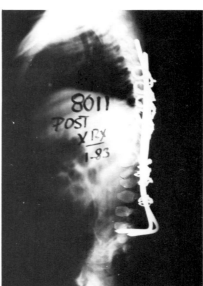

Fig. 6-8*C*.

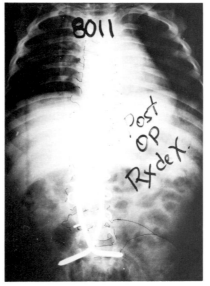

Fig. 6-8*D*.

Fig. 6-8*E*.

The known infection rate associated with SSI is less than 4%. At the Mexico City Shriners' Hospital, there have been two deep infections, for which it was necessary to remove all the material and treat the patient with external plaster and polypropylene casts. There has been one death—a ten-year-old patient with a 110°

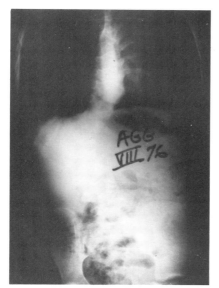 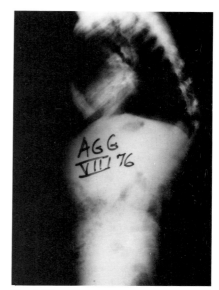

Fig. 6-9*A* and *B*. AP and lateral x-ray of a congenital thoracolumbar scoliosis with a long dorsal kyphosis.

Fig. 6-9*B*.

rigid lumbar kyphosis and a 35% vital capacity restriction, who suffered a cardiac arrest during posterior approach surgery to resect the kyphosis.

Thirteen cases have evolved satisfactorily, with an average loss of correction of 15° in two years without external support in ten cases, and with Risser antigravity casts used for four months in three cases (Fig. 6-8).

Conclusions

The principal advantage of SSI vis-à-vis other techniques is the possibility of not having to use external supports, and of avoiding prolonged bed rest. The latter is particularly important in these patients, since it facilitates urologic treatment, treatment of pressure sores, rehabilitation, and reconstructive surgery. SSI reduces the risk of pseudarthrosis by providing a greater internal fixation. The psychologic impact on the patient and his family is highly encouraging, since the patient requires no external support and has a great enthusiasm for his rehabilitation.

Editor's Commentary

In the treatment of paralytic scoliosis, two aspects have to be considered: One is stability of the spine and the other is correction of the deformity. This is true for

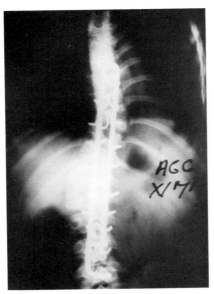

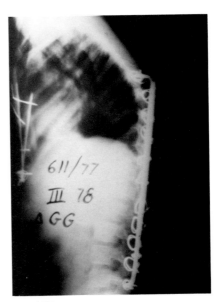

C and *D*, AP and lateral x-rays of patient in Fig. 1*A*, well covered in the scoliotic area with the instrumentation. The lateral film shows pectus excavatum and a short instrumentation area in the cephalic part of the kyphotic deformity.

Fig. 6-9*D*.

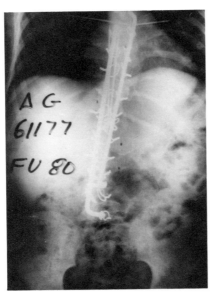

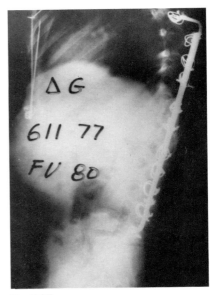

E and *F*, AP x-ray shows good maintenance of correction. The lateral film shows increased deformity due to lack of cephalad fixation.

Fig. 6-9*F*.

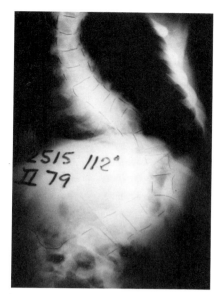 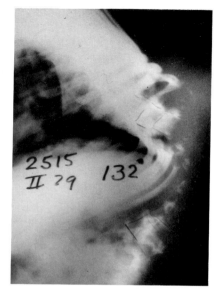

Fig. 6-10*A* and *B*. Seventeen-year-old male post-poliomyelitis with a thoracolumbar curve of 112° and a thoracolumbar kyphosis of 132°. He also has pelvic obliquity and an arthrodesis.

Fig. 6-10*B*.

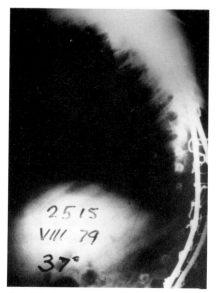 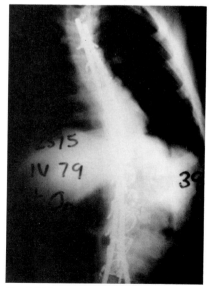

C and *D*, Same patient as Fig. 2*A*. Scoliosis, corrected to 39°, is well balanced. The lateral is corrected to 37° of thoracolumbar kyphosis.

Fig. 6-10*D*.

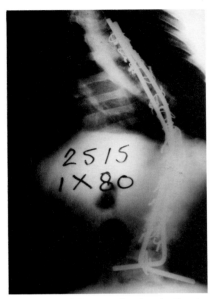 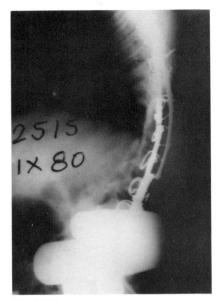

E and *F*, AP follow-up of patient in Fig. 2*A*. Fractured rods, loss of correction, loss of balance, and pseudarthrosis occurred. Lateral film shows fractured bars and loss of correction.

Fig. 6-10*F.*

both adults and growing children. Producing *stability* means maintaining instrumentation of a spine as long as is necessary to produce an erect patient. *Correction* of the spine means performing instrumentation of the spine to avoid progression of the deformity and balancing the deformity to improve the way of life of the patient.

Sometimes even with paralytic curves, compensatory curves need not undergo instrumentation if they are in an area of good muscle balance, provide compensatory curves for residual deformity, and are in themselves stable. If no compensatory curves exist after correcting scoliosis, one should build them into the SSI system above and below the newly corrected deformity to equal the residual deformity.

One frequent mistake is not continuing instrumentation far enough into the dorsal kyphosis, especially when this is structural and nonreducible. This brings about progressive deformity (Fig. 6-9).

There are two other deformities in paralytic scoliosis that have in the past been responsible for most of our failures: pelvic obliquity and thoracodorsal kyphosis (Fig. 6-10). Both these deformities must be reduced completely before the spine undergoes instrumentation (elongation of soft tissues and shortening procedures). Dwyer and Selkie procedures are very effective in the thoracic and upper lumbar spine, but there are two major inconveniences. First, the segmental vessels must be ligated over the entire area of instrumentation; second, they produce an essentially flat back.

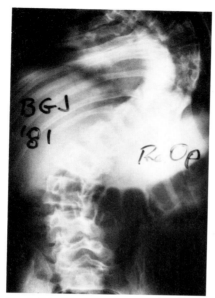

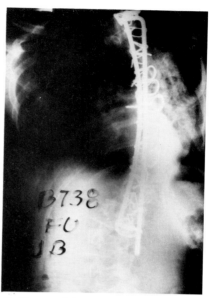

Fig. 6-11A. AP x-ray of male, age 17 years, showing post-poliomyelitis sequelae with a thoracic scoliosis of 115° and a 75° rotation by CAT scan.

B, AP x-ray of the same patient as in Fig. 3A, postoperatively corrected to 53° after three-level vertebrectomy, six-level diskectomy, and 40° vertebral transposition to the midline of the body.

If SSI is contemplated as a second procedure, a second vascular insult will be provoked by the procedure, which makes the danger of an ischemic cord more probable. Obviously, the second problem is that molding the physiologic axial curves becomes impossible. In growing children, I believe that it has been well shown that subperiosteal dissection does not necessarily lead to arthrodesis. Enough fixation should be done to produce a balanced correction and stability of the spine.[38,39]

In very severe deformities, spot, anterior (possibly even a vertebrectomy) or posterior fusion to align the spine, without arthrodesis, might be necessary within a much more extensive SSI. Rotational deformities of the thorax in paralytics are very important because of the thoracic cage deformity (Fig. 6-11). Unfortunately, to correct rotation, diskectomies must be done, as well as resection of the concave ribs and release of the convex transverse process. This produces a transposition of the vertebral column toward the midline. One wonders if so much surgery in a delicate patient is justified and if it is going to help his breathing. On the other hand, correction and fixation in conditions that we know will produce a progressive deformity, like muscular dystrophy and myelodysplasia, would be done at an early age, before the production of severe deformity.

Pelvic fixation is extremely important in these cases and must be individualized. The Galveston technique is the most exacting surgically and probably the most rigid in patients with bad bone substance in the iliac crests. Transiliac fixation is the easiest to perform and provides good fixation for correcting or producing lordosis.

References

1. Allen BL, Ferguson RC: The Galveston technique for L rod instrumentation of the scoliotic spine. Spine 7:276-284, 1982.

2. Bergofsky EH, Turino GM, Fishman AP: Cardiorespiratory failure in kyphoscoliosis. Medicine 38:263, 1959.

3. Block AJ, Wexler J, McDonnell EJ: Cardiopulmonary failure of the hunchback: A possible therapeutic approach. JAMA 212:1520, 1970.

4. Blount WP, Moe JH: The Milwaukee Brace. Baltimore, MD, Williams and Wilkins Co., 1973.

5. Cardoso MA: Sociedad Mexicana de Ortopedia. Escoliosis en el Hospital Shriners. Análisis de 425 casos (1962-1974). México 1974.

6. Cardoso MA, Luque RE: Osteotomias de columna. Anales de Ortopedia y Traumatología 12:2, Abril-Junio, 1976.

7. Cardoso MA, Luque RE: Instrumentation segmentaria. Desarrollo de una técnica. Anales de Ortopedia y Traumatología 14:2, 1978.

8. Caro CG, Dubois AB: Pulmonary function in kyphoscoliosis. Thorax 16:282, 1961.

9. Dwyer AF: Experience of anterior correction of scoliosis. Clin Ortho 93:191-206, 1973.

10. Godfrey S: Respiratory and cardiovascular consequences of scoliosis. Respiration 27:67, 1970.

11. Goldstein LA: Terminology committee report. Scoliosis Research Society, Fourth Annual Meeting, Los Angeles, CA, 1969.

12. Goldstein LA, Waugh TR: Classification and terminology of scoliosis. Clin Ortho 93:10-22, 1973.

13. Hall J: Remarks on spine deformity in myelomeningocele. Scoliosis Research Society, Wilmington, DE, 1972.

14. Hensinger RN, MacEwen DG: Spinal deformity associated with heritable neurological conditions: Spinal muscular atrophy, Friedreich's ataxia, familial dysautonomia and Charcot-Marie-Tooth disease. J Bone Jt Surg 58A:13-23, 1976.

15. Herring JA, Wenger DR: S.S.I., a preliminary report of 40 consecutive cases. Spine 7(3):285-298, 1982.

16. Johnson BE, Westgate HD: Methods of predicting vital capacity in patients with thoracic scoliosis. J Bone Jt Surg 52A:14-33, 1970.

17. Luque ER, Cardoso AM: Sequential correction of scoliosis with rigid internal fixation. Ortho Trans 1:136, 1977.

18. Luque ER, Cardoso MA: Treatment of scoliosis without arthrodesis or external support. (Preliminary Report). Ortho Trans 1:37-38, 1977.

19. Luque ER, Cardoso MA: Segmental correction of scoliosis with rigid internal fixation. Scoliosis Research Society, Ottawa, Ontario, Canada, 1976.

20. Luque ER, Cardoso MA: Segmental correction and fixation of the spine, Exhibit at 45th Annual Meeting of the Amer Acad Ortho Surg, Dallas, TX, 1978.

21. Luque ER: Paralytic scoliosis in growing children. Clin Ortho 163:202-210, 1982.

22. MacEwen GD: Report of the morbidity committee. Scoliosis Research Society, Hartford, CT, 1971.

23. Makley JT, Herndon CH, Inkley S, Doershuk C, Matthews LW, Post RH, Littell AS: Pulmonary function in paralytic and non-paralytic scoliosis before and after treatment. A study of sixty-three cases. J Bone Jt Surg 50A:1379, 1968.

24. Mayfield JK: Severe spine deformity in myelodysplasia and sacral agenesis. Spine 6(5):498-509, 1981.

25. Moe JH: Management of paralytic scoliosis. S Med J 50:67-81, 1957.

26. Nachemson A: A long term follow-up study of non-treated scoliosis. Acta Ortho Scand 39:466-476, 1968.

27. O'Brien JP: Anterior and posterior correction and fusion for paralytic scoliosis. Clin Ortho 86:151-153, 1972.

28. Raycroft JH, Curtis BH: Spinal curvature in myelomeningocele: Natural history and etiology. In AAOS Symposium on Myelomeningocele, Hartford, CT, 1970. St. Louis, C.V. Mosby Co., 1972.

29. Romero JJ: Correccion quirurgica de la escoliosis en niños con fijacion segmentaria tecnica Dr. Luque. Tesis Hospital Shriners, México, 1981.

30. Sharrard WJW: Spinal osteotomy for congenital kyphosis in myelomeningocele. J Bone Jt Surg 50B:466-471, 1968.

31. Sriran K, Bobechko WP, Hall JE: Surgical management of spinal deformities in spina bifida. J Bone Jt Surg 54B:666-676, 1972.

32. Sullivan AJ, Conner SB: Comparison of Harrington instrumentation and segmental spinal instrumentation in the management of neuromuscular spinal deformity. Spine 7(3):299-304, 1982.

33. Taddonio RF: Segmental spinal instrumentation in the management of neuromuscular spinal deformity. Spine 7(3):305-311, 1982.

34. Winter RB: Congenital kyphosis. J Bone Jt Surg 55A:223-256, 1973.

35. Winter RB: Congenital kyphosis. Clin Ortho 128:26-32, 1977.

36. Winter RB, Hall JE: Kyphosis in childhood and adolescence. Spine 3:285-308, 1978.

37. Wilkins KE, Gibson DA: The patterns of spinal deformity in Duchenne muscular dystrophy. J Bone Jt Surg 58A:24-36, 1976.

38. Luque ER: Paralytic scoliosis in growing children. Clin Ortho 163:202-209, March 1982.

39. McAfe, PC, Lubicky JP, Werner F: The use of S.S.I. to preserve longitudinal rod. An experimental study. J Bone Jt Surg 85a(7):935-942, September 1983.

Segmental Spinal Instrumentation in Idiopathic Scoliosis

7

SINCE THE INTRODUCTION OF SEGMENTAL spinal instrumentation (SSI), numerous authors have advocated it for the treatment of various spinal deformities.[1,6,8,9] However, in all but a few centers, a gray area has existed in regard to the treatment of idiopathic scoliosis. While it has been shown by biomechanical testing that segmental spinal instrumentation offers superior fixation as compared with Harrington instrumentation, concern has been voiced over the safety of sublaminar wiring.[10,11] For this reason, many have felt that the presumed added risk of sublaminar wiring was offset by the benefit in neurogenic cases, while the potential risk in idiopathic cases was felt to be too great to employ SSI as the standard means of treatment.

Other concerns have also been voiced. Since the operation seemed to be more involved than similar procedures, it would follow that the operating time would be prolonged. If this were the case, would the blood loss then be greater and other factors regarding morbidity be higher? For example, might one expect to see increased postoperative pulmonary complications with atelectasis? Would blood loss be greater?

TABLE 7-1.

100% Females	— Idiopathic Scoliosis
80% Males	— Idiopathic Scoliosis
20% Males	— Kyphosis

TABLE 7-2.

	Harrington Rods	Luque Rods
Age Detected	13	13
Age Fused	14.9	14.8
Levels Fused	9.5 Vertebrae	10.5 Vertebrae

In addition to the concern about increased morbidity, other factors were felt to be important in evaluating the efficacy of the procedure in idiopathic scoliosis. Curve correction and maintenance of correction as well as time in hospital were chief among them.

It has been argued that postoperative casting and bracing are not such heinous treatments that their use should be condemned. However, many patients when confronted with this prospect have chosen not to undergo surgical correction for their deformities because of prolonged immobilization.

Harrington vs SSI

To evaluate the issues brought forth by this discussion, it was decided by one of the authors (AK) to do a study comparing Harrington instrumentation with segmental spinal instrumentation. The study consisted of 42 patients who were treated consecutively with either Harrington instrumentation or segmental spinal instrumentation. All individuals were in the adolescent age range and had either idiopathic scoliosis or Scheuermann's kyphosis. As can be seen in Table 7-1, all the females had idiopathic adolescent scoliosis, while 80% of the males had idiopathic scoliosis. The average age at which the children had fusions is presented

TABLE 7-3.

	HARRINGTON RODS	LUQUE RODS
Hypotensive anesthesia	84%	100%
Blood loss	1801 cc	1450 cc

TABLE 7-4.

	HARRINGTON RODS	LUQUE RODS
Operative Time	3.07 Hours	3.2 Hours
Length of Hospitalization	12.5 Days	10.5 Days

in Table 7-2. The age ranges were essentially identical. The number of levels fused was also quite similar.

The operative technique utilized for segmental spinal instrumentation was the same as presented by Luque et al.[1,6] The Harrington cases used Harrington distraction-compression instrumentation with a transverse loading device. Up to the point of instrumentation, operative technique was identical. All patients underwent surgery on a Hall-Relton frame, and hypotensive anesthesia was used. Eighty-four percent of the patients receiving Harrington instrumentation were operated on under a hypotensive technique, while 100% of the Luque cases were done under hypotension. Technical difficulties in obtaining arterial catheterization accounted for lack of complete compliance in the use of hypotension. Otherwise, the operative technique was completely standard, utilizing a subperiosteal dissection, complete cleaning of posterior elements, and facet fusion. All cases were grafted with iliac bone in addition to local bone.

Results of Study

Results of the study, analyzed two years postoperatively, are presented in Tables 7-3 through 7-6. From Table 7-3, it is apparent that blood loss was not greater with segmental spinal instrumentation. The fact that the blood loss was less and the amount of blood that had to be replaced was less might be related to the difficulty

TABLE 7-5.

Curve Correction	Harrington Rods	Luque Rods
At 6 Weeks	40%	30%
At Longest Follow-up	29%	33%
Follow-up	19 Months	18.5 Months

TABLE 7-6.

Postoperative Complications	Harrington Rods	Luque Rods
Urinary Retention	32%	58%
Gastrointestinal	23%	29%
Neurologic	0%*	0%
Pseudarthrosis	0%	0%
Instrument Failure	0%	0%
Dural Laceration	0%	0%
Progression Beyond Instrumentation	0%	5%
Rod Rotation	0%	10%
Wire Breakage	0%	5%

*3 Patients from SSI group had lateral femoral cutaneous nerve palsy.

with hypotensive anesthesia described previously for two of the Harrington cases. Table 7-4 shows that the operative time was slightly prolonged with Luque instrumentation. There was approximately a 20-minute difference in average operative time between the two procedures. On the other hand, the length of hospitalization was a full two days less for the SSI patients.

Curve correction with the two procedures can be seen in Table 7-5. It is apparent that in this series, Harrington instrumentation provided a better initial correction but a greater loss of correction at follow-up. Only 3% loss of correction was noted in the Luque group, while an 11% loss of correction was noted in the Harrington group. All individuals with Harrington instrumentation were treated postoperatively for six months with a Kosair spinal orthosis, while the patients treated with SSI had no form of external immobilization postoperatively.

Table 7-6 is a summary of complications encountered during the study. Of particular note is the fact there were no significant neurologic complications.

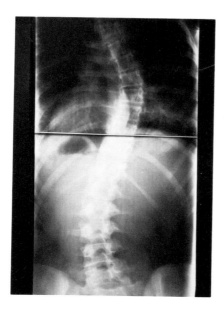

Fig. 7-1A. This 13-year-old, who had a 40° right thoracic curve preoperatively, is shown at six weeks and at 14 months follow-up. *B,* At six weeks, the curve measured 32°. At the three-month check-up, the rod was noted to have displaced subsequent to wire breakage. *C,* The follow-up x-ray at 14 months showed no further loss of correction than that noted at three months. Final Cobb angle measurement is 38°.

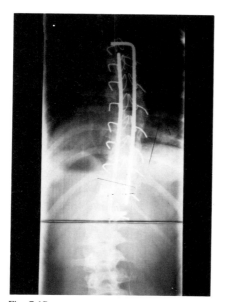

Fig. 7-1*B.*

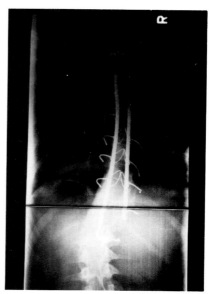

Fig. 7-1*C.*

Passage of the sublaminar wires did not produce dural lacerations or other neurologic problems. The most significant complication in this group was wire breakage, with some subsequent loss of correction.

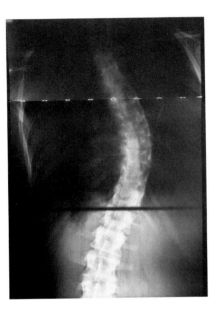

Fig. 7-2A. Thirty-year-old female with a preoperative right thoracic curve of 49° from T6 to T12. *B,* Six weeks after SSI, the Cobb angle is 26°. *C,* At five-month follow-up, a broken wire is noted at T4 with no subsequent loss of correction.

Treatment of Idiopathic Scoliosis

Buoyed by the initial success with idiopathic adolescent cases and by the results of our study, we treated the patients subsequently presenting with idiopathic scoliosis in all age groups with segmental spinal instrumentation (Figs. 7-1 and 7-2). Our results to this point have been gratifying. Table 7-7 presents the average ages of the patients when the curves were detected and the average ages at which they were fused. The number of levels fused is also presented. Sex distribution is as expected, with a preponderance of females. There have been 81 cases of idiopathic scoliosis of both the adult and adolescent variety that have been treated with this technique.

Pulmonary function tests were routinely obtained preoperatively (Table 7-8). None of the patients had severe obstructive or restrictive lung disease. As might be expected, the adolescent group had predominantly normal lung functions, while the adult group had a preponderance of mild or moderate obstructive or restrictive disease.

Our routine for the past five years has included autotransfusion. Since many of our patients do not live near the hospital, an attempt has not been made to save blood over a long period; rather, the patient has one unit of his own blood withdrawn the day before surgery. Volume replacement is accomplished with one liter of Ringer's lactate. In patients weighing less than 100 pounds, the amount of blood taken is reduced proportionate to stature.

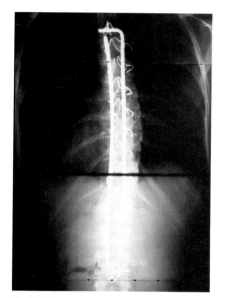

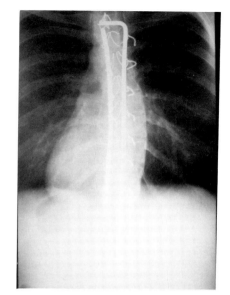

Fig. 7-2B.   Fig. 7-2C.

TABLE 7-7.

	ADULTS	ADOLESCENTS
Age Detected	17	11.6
Age Fused	30	14
Levels Fused	10	10.5
Females	43 or 88%	24 or 75%
Males	6 or 12%	8 or 25%

TABLE 7-8.

PULMONARY FUNCTIONS	ADULTS	ADOLESCENTS
Within Normal Limits	16 or 33%	19 or 59%
Mild Obstructive/Restrictive	24 or 49%	8 or 25%
Moderate Obstructive/Restrictive	4 or 8%	3 or 9%
No Result Reported	5 or 10%	2 or 6%

TABLE 7-9.

	ADULTS	ADOLESCENTS
Preop Hematocrit	42	42.9
Discharge Hematocrit	33	33
Blood Replacement	2.6 Units	2 Units
(1 unit being auto)	33 or 67%	25 or 78%
Hypotensive Anesthesia	47 or 96% Nipride	100% Nipride
Blood Loss	1598 cc	1448 cc

TABLE 7-10.

	ADULTS	ADOLESCENTS
Operative Time	3.5 Hours	3 Hours

As can be seen in Table 7-9, our blood loss averages 1.5 units in both the adult and the adolescent populations. The number of patients receiving one unit of their own blood back is presented. All patients were discharged with a hematocrit of greater than 30%.

As might be expected, operative time was somewhat longer for adults than for adolescents (Table 7-10). One half-hour more was required to clean the posterior elements in the adults. It might also be added that frequently the ligamentum flavum was calcified in the adult population, requiring extra care in removing it. In some cases, the calcification was significant enough to require the use of a bur or other power equipment to facilitate the procedure.

As a rule, it took an extra day for the adult patients to get out of the hospital, as compared with the adolescents (Table 7-11). Most patients were walking on the fifth or sixth postoperative day. Once peristalsis was established, most patients felt well enough to get up to go to the bathroom and to walk in the hall.

Complications

Postoperative complications were divided into immediate and long-term varieties. As presented in Table 7-12, the most common complication was urinary retention. There were no major neurologic complications. Not included in the table were

TABLE 7-11.

	ADULTS	ADOLESCENTS
Postop Day of Discharge	9 Days	8 Days

TABLE 7-12.

IMMEDIATE POSTOP COMPLICATIONS	ADULTS	ADOLESCENTS
None	10 or 20%	6 or 19%
Urinary Retention	36 or 73%	21 or 66%
G.I.	3 or 6%	6 or 19%
Neurologic	6 or 12%	3 or 9%
Vaginal Infection	1 or 2%	2 or 6%
Transfusion Reaction	3 or 6%	1 or 3%

transient lateral femoral cutaneous nerve palsy caused by the positioning on the operating table or cluneal nerve palsies caused by overzealous retraction in obtaining bone graft. Of the three patients with neurologic complications, two had painful dysesthesias in the leg and foot, and one adolescent had what seemed to be a very mild S1 motor weakness that gradually improved postoperatively from the time it was noted until it cleared in four days. The transfusion reactions were all minor, consisting of a rash, fever, or both.

Long-term complications are listed in Table 7-13. Approximately one-third of the patients in both groups had some type of long-term complication. The most common problem has been instrument failure. There have been no cases of rod failure, but 16 cases of wire breakage. Most of these have occurred within the first 90 days postoperatively. Of these, eight adults and one adolescent have required reoperation. In two of the adults, all instrumentation was removed. In the remainder of the patients, only the rod tip or the broken wire, or both, was removed. None of the instrumentation was removed prior to healing of the bone graft. No case of dislocation of the rod was significant enough in the early phases of fusion to require reoperation.

Late pain has also been a feature of instrumentation (Fig. 7-3). Most of the discomfort has been a result of irritation by either the rod tip or the wire. Four patients have been reoperated for pain syndromes without instrument failure. In

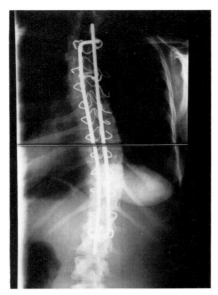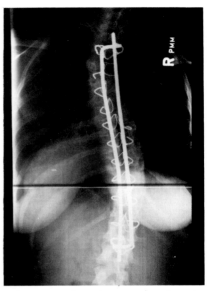

Fig. 7-3A. Twenty-seven-year-old with a pre-operative 58° left high thoracic curve and 48° right lower thoracic curve. Postoperatively, her curves measure 42° and 33°. This correction was maintained well, but at 26 months, (B) the patient had persistent interscapular pain on the right, and the sublaminar wires were subsequently removed in the area of discomfort. Her symptoms resolved subsequently.

these cases, the offending wire was removed or shortened and rebent so as to avoid irritating the soft tissues. No cases of pseudarthrosis have been proven to this point. Two cases of pseudarthrosis are suspected in adults. Only one patient had long-term neurologic difficulties; this was a case of persistent radicular pain, which has not cleared in spite of removal of instrumentation.

Results

In Table 7-14, the amount of curve correction is presented. It can be seen that the average adult correction in idiopathic scoliosis was 25% in adults and 30% in adolescents. Only a 2° loss of correction was seen in both groups. Average follow-up in the adult group was 12 months, while in the adolescent group it was 11 months.

The results obtained with segmental spinal instrumentation in idiopathic scoliosis do not seem as good with regard to percentage of correction as the results with Harrington instrumentation presented in the literature.[1,6] However, in our own series, the amount of correction seems to be similar. It must be remembered that both systems of instrumentation are quite powerful. Both certainly have the potential to cause neurologic embarrassment, and for this reason great care should

TABLE 7-13.

Long-Term Complications	Adults	Adolescents
Pain	9 or 18%	4 or 12.5%
Instrumentation Failure (rotation, breakage)	10 or 20%	6 or 19%
Hardware Removed	8 or 16%	1 or 3%
Seroma	1 or 2%	3 or 9%
Neurologic	1 or 2%	—
Pseudarthrosis	0	0
None	33 or 67%	21 or 66%

TABLE 7-14.

Curves	Adults	Adolescents
Preop	49°	40°
At 6 Weeks Check-up	37°	28°
At Longest Follow-up	35°	30°
Average Follow-up	12 Months	11 Months

be taken when using them. In his presentations, Luque has stressed the importance of balancing the spine. The three-dimensional concept of spinal stability that he has emphasized should be kept in mind when doing any type of spinal surgery for spinal deformity. It has been this tenet that has been used in our center. Attempting to correct the curvature to a greater degree than can be obtained on bending or traction films has not been done on our patients. It is this fact that most likely accounts for the paucity of neurologic complications.

The materials and methods used in segmental spinal instrumentation are still evolving. Early wire breakage in our cases has been, for the most part, secondary to not contouring the rod precisely to the spine. When there has been technical difficulty in obtaining precise contouring, the wires have been noted to break more easily. Allen and Ferguson have discussed this problem and have recommended double wiring at the extremes of the instrumentation. (See Chap. 9.) In our experience, this has not been a uniformly successful solution. Vitalium rods and wires have been introduced as a result of the work done in Galveston. This system is currently being evaluated.

Until the institution of the vitalium L-rod instrumentation, all adults were

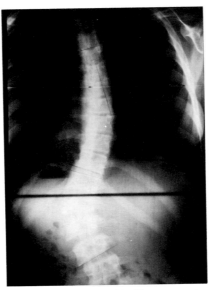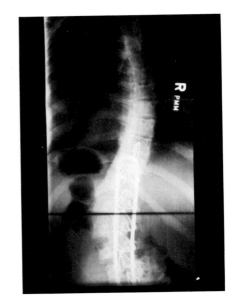

Fig. 7-4*A*. Twelve-year-old with a progressive left lumbar curve of 45° convexed left from T12 to L3. Her postoperative Cobb angle measurement was 33° (*B*).

fused with at least one 1/4-inch rod. In the thoracic spine, frequently one 3/16-inch rod and one 1/4-inch rod would be utilized. In double major curves or in lumbar curves, two 1/4-inch rods were utilized. The vitalium system currently offers only the 3/15-inch rod, and the manufacturer feels that a 1/4-inch rod will not be necessary because of the apparent strength of the smaller device.

If growth is anticipated, a double L-rod system is still utilized. While several authors feel that fusion stops spinal growth, it has been shown by Luque that growth does continue after SSI and fusion.[2,4,5,7] With the double L-rod system, the spine is not tethered. It is hoped that growth can continue as a result without further deformity. In cases in which growth has ceased, rectangular rods are being utilized if possible. These rods will not dislocate as easily and have greater torsional stiffness.

Segmental fixation has provided the means to treat thoracic lordosis (Fig. 7-4). Because the spine is segmentally fixed, it has been possible to improve this deformity.

It has not been possible in our experience to generate normal postural curves with the correction of scoliosis. However, segmental spinal instrumentation has allowed for the production of more normal curve patterns (Fig. 7-5). Wire breakage has been a problem when correction of pathologic curves is attempted beyond that which is easily obtainable at the operating table. This is true for both postural, scoliotic, and kyphotic deformities.

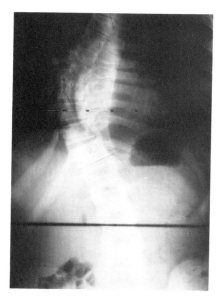

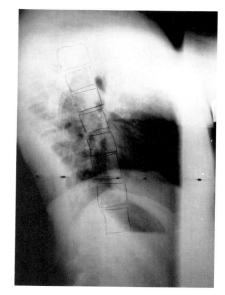

Fig. 7-5*A* and *B*. Fifteen-year-old boy with a −10° kyphosis from T5 to T12 associated with a 47° scoliosis convexed right from T6 to T12. *C* and *D*, Postoperatively, the hypokyphosis has been converted to a kyphosis of 15°, and his scoliosis is 30° by Cobb measurement.

Fig. 7-5B.

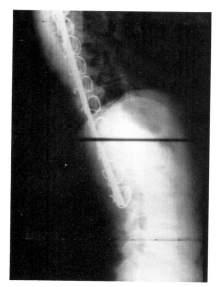

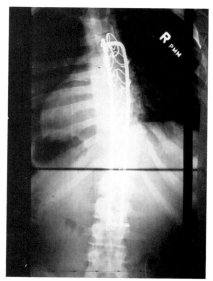

Fig. 7-5*C*.

Fig. 7-5*D*.

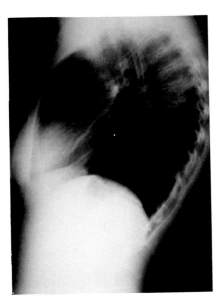

Fig. 7-6A. Twenty-one-year-old with a 72° kyphosis from T3 to T12. Postoperative x-rays at six weeks (B) and at six months (C) show no loss of correction at 50°; however, there has been wire breakage at L2.

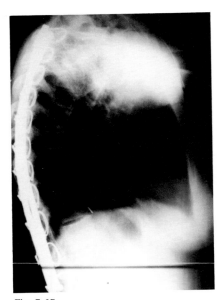

Fig. 7-6B.

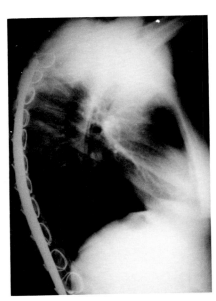

Fig. 7-6C.

One drawback of segmental spinal instrumentation in idiopathic scoliosis is the lack of derotation that occurs with instrumentation (Fig. 7-6). Without a distraction force, derotation does not seem to be as great. This is of consequence from a cosmetic point of view. Luque has advocated sectioning of the ribs on the concavity of the curve. In his experience, the results have been gratifying. This technique has not been used in our center.

Conclusion

Surgical correction of idiopathic scoliosis is a procedure that should be carried out by those familiar with current concepts and who have broad experience in spinal surgery. Surgeons who are thoughtful and well-trained in the treatment of spinal deformity should be able to add segmental spinal instrumentation to their armamentarium of procedures without fear that it is particularly risky from a neurologic standpoint. Because the procedure does require that the surgeon deal with the spinal canal and its content, it cannot be recommended for use by those who are occasional scoliologists. However, it does seem that when the technique is properly applied, the results justify its use.

There can be no question that this population of patients is much happier when handled without external forms of immobilization. The freedom obtained and the early return to normal activities that has been experienced by this population have made it the standard treatment for the patients in our center with idiopathic scoliosis.

The final justification for the use of segmental spinal instrumentation in idiopathic scoliosis is economic. It has been possible for us to discharge patients from the hospital a minimum of two days earlier than patients who were treated by the Harrington technique. This has allowed a 15% to 20% savings in hospitalization cost, making the procedure cost-effective as well.

Editor's Commentary

The coauthors compared two series of patients: one treated with pure Harrington instrumentation and the other with pure SSI. There was no chance of complications. This represents a normal, accepted surgical group of idiopathic scoliotic patients. The only difference was that the Harrington group had six months of external immobilization, and the patients treated with SSI had no external immobilization. No effort was made to obtain maximum correction; the aim was a balanced spine. The surgical time was increased by 20 minutes in the SSI patients, yet the blood loss was roughly equal. Postural curves were conserved with greater ease in SSI patients. Derotation was considered a nonsolved problem.

Does elongation by distraction produce an apparently lesser hump, or does it promote progressive deterioration of vital capacity?

In spite of no external immobilization and less initial correction, the SSI group had a better end result as measured by the Cobb angle. As reported, the patients seem to be happier. The question remains, in the long run, is a well-balanced patient with an arthrodesis better off than a distracted patient with a straight back? What will be the effect of sublaminar wiring? Why is posterior laminar fusion reported to produce stenosis of the canal, only present in the lumbar region? (Was it there at the start?) Ultimately, are patients with 40° balanced curves better off without arthrodesis? Physiologically, what is the most important question: Deformity? Age? Longevity? All are transient.

I feel that in a deformed patient, his immediate future lifestyle is more important that his long-term history, especially at the present stage of our knowledge. We are not sure what the natural course of spinal deformity is. We are only sure that we have made formidable advances in understanding and solving spinal pathology and biomechanics. Ten more years of knowledge will probably lead to better care of the arthrodesed patient, in relation to what we already know about untreated patients.

References

1. Allen BL Jr: The Galveston technique for L-rod instrumentation of the scoliotic spine. Spine Vol. 7, No. 3, 1982.

2. Haas SL: Influence of fusion of the spine on growth of the vertebrae. Arch Surg 41:607, 1940.

3. Harrington PR: Correction and internal fixation by spinal instrumentation. J Bone Jt Surg 44A:591, June 1962.

4. Johnson JTH, Southwick WO: Bone growth after spine fusion. J Bone Jt Surg 42A:1396, 1960.

5. Letts RM, Bobechko WP: Fusion of the scoliotic spine in young children. Clin Ortho 101:136-145, 1974.

6. Luque ER: The correction of postural curves of the spine. Spine Vol. 7, No. 3, 1982.

7. Moe JH, Sundberg AB, Gustilo R: A clinical study of spine fusion in the growing child. J Bone Jt Surg 46B:784-785, 1964.

8. Sullivan JA, Conner SB: Comparison of Harrington instrumentation in the management of neuromuscular spinal deformity. Spine Vol. 7, No. 3, 1982.

9. Taddonio RF: Segmental spinal instrumentation in the management of neuromuscular spinal deformity. Spine Vol. 7, No. 3, 1982.

10. Wenger DR, Carollo JJ, Wilkerson JA Jr: Biomechanics of scoliosis correction by segmental spinal instrumentation. Spine Vol. 7, No. 3, 1982.

11. Wenger DR, Carollo JJ, Wilkerson JA Jr, Wauters K, Herring JA: Laboratory testing of segmental spinal instrumentation versus traditional Harrington instrumentation for scoliosis treatment. Spine Vol. 7, No. 3, 1982.

12. Winter RB: Scoliosis and spinal growth. Ortho Rev Vol. VI, No. 7, July, 1977.

A Clinical Assessment of 357 Cases of Segmental Spinal Instrumentation

8

DESPITE OUR CONSERVATIVE BUT ENTHUSIASTIC beginning with the SSI program in 1981, we have reached a point in time at which we believe we can present a critical review of our material, which we hope will be helpful to the learning spine surgeon.

This chapter is divided into two parts. The first presents our learning experiences and changes in our techniques that we felt were necessary to gain better results. In the second part of this chapter, we review an additional 216 cases, which we call the second phase of our SSI study.

In the first 141 cases in our center, we employed the Luque technique as presented to us—double-L rod segmental spinal instrumentation (SSI). The average follow-up was 16.24 months. It was quite obvious that segmental spinal instrumentation was an excellent means of obtaining spinal stability and had the reported benefit of needing no postoperative immobilization.

There were two perioperative deaths. The remaining 139 patients were evalu-

TABLE 8-1

Idiopathic—15 Cases

Adolescent—4
   1 redo with kyphosis below previous fusion
   1 thoracic hypokyphotic
Adult—7
   No previous surgery
Juvenile—4
   1 redo from juvenile Leatherman rods
Combined with anterior procedure—4
   2 adult diskectomies (adult Marfan)
   2 juvenile diskectomies
Trolley—1
Braced—11
Not braced—4
Estimated blood loss—1064.33 cc/case
   1090.00 cc/case—adult and adolescent
    993.75 cc/case—juvenile
     50.00 cc/case—Luque Trolley
Percentage of correction—scoliosis
   52.90%—adult
   47.80%—adolescent
   61.00%—juvenile
Percentage of correction—kyphosis
   34.40%—adult
   42.00%—juvenile
Operating time
   4.81 hours—adult and adolescent
   4.50 hours—juvenile
   1.70 hours—Luque Trolley
Complications—1
   1 adolescent—broken wire, no bracing
Percentage of complications—6.70%

---

ated for evidence of metal failure or pseudarthrosis. Lower spine (T12 to the sacrum) posterior fusions were found to have a significantly greater failure rate if not braced than other procedures. Our technique was not altered appreciably in the early months. Our indications for the Luque procedure were the following: neuromuscular disorders, paralytic collapsing spines, osteoporosis, osteogenesis imperfecta, paraplegic spinal cord injuries, sensory defects as in myelodysplasia, degenerative lumbosacral lesions, and spondylolisthesis.

In the first group, our complication rate has been high. We have seen one case of temporary paralysis; a number of infected wounds, both superficial and deep, that have required late removal of the instrumentation; and a number of superficial infections that healed in time. There have been three cases of pseudarthrosis.

The greatest deviations from the original Luque program have been the use of a postoperative brace, and doing many more anterior procedures to give greater stability to the collapsing or unstable spine. We have used a simple Louisville

TABLE 8-2

Congenital—15 Cases

2 redo
4 Luque Trolleys
Combined with anterior procedure—11
    8 excision of hemivertebrae
    3 multiple diskectomies
Braced—10
    2 crutch-type spine brace
    7 Kosair Scoliosis Orthosis
    1 plastic-type brace
Not braced—5
    1 placed in brace two months after surgery for increased kyphosis
    2 placed on bed rest
Estimated blood loss—635.70 cc/case
    120.00 cc/case—Luque Trolley
Percentage of correction
    33.67%—scoliosis
    37.40%—kyphosis
Operating time
    3.95 hours—per case
Complications—4
    Wound dehiscence
    Wound infection—staph with prominent wires
    Right foot paresis and hyperesthesia—resolved
    Paraplegia—late recovery (6 months)

Kosair crutch-type spine brace postoperatively in correction of kyphosis and in some of the paralytic disorders for which we felt greater protection was necessary. We have also used the brace in fracture cases and have felt that bracing minimized the patient's pain and general discomfort. In reviewing our cases, we have found no rod breakage or wire breakage in the cases that were braced.

We have always felt very strongly that many anterior fusions and areas of anterior stabilization should be established in the paralytic and weakened spine in a two-stage procedure in order to give better and, it is hoped, lasting stability. These are producing our best clinical and functional results.

In the second phase of our study, we altered our original surgical techniques. We have tended to use the double-L rods in fewer cases, have increased the indications, and yet have been more selective in these cases. With better selection of cases, we have had fewer complications and have continued to gain experience. We have used longer rods as well as replacing the double-L rods with rectangular ones. Smaller diameter rods have been sufficient in many cases, particularly for those in which we have done anterior stabilization. The indications for bracing have remained the same.

Fascinated with the potential for growth using Luque instrumentation without fusion, we have carefully selected a number of congenital scoliosis cases for spinal instrumentation without fusion after vertebral body resection and discectomies (Luque Trolley). With this technique, we are altering the forces of growth as well as the direction.

Part I

Of the 141 patients reviewed, 79 underwent posterior procedures, and 62 were combined with anterior procedures. The anterior procedures comprised the following:

Multiple diskectomies	29
Disks with vertebrectomies	2
Vertebrectomies	19
Zielke	10
Tumors	1
Disks and screws	1

The complications were frequent considering the type of patient. There were four judgment errors. There were no instrument failures when combined with the use of the brace. A total of 61 braces were used.

The diagnoses are analyzed in Tables 8-1 to 8-14.

There were 16 uncategorized cases. Table 8-15 is a summary of complications encountered.

Part II

Since 1981, 357 segmental spinal instrumentations have been performed at Norton Kosair-Children's Hospitals in Louisville, Kentucky. Part I of this chapter analyzed the first 141 cases—the techniques used to perform the procedures, complications that have accompanied these procedures, and the overall results that have been obtained. Part II is an analysis of the last 216 segmental spinal instrumentations and a look at their early results. Technical changes and variations in approach, using these techniques, were made based upon the results gained from the earlier group.

This group of patients had degenerative lumbar disease, fractures, Scheuermann's kyphosis, idiopathic scoliosis, congenital scoliosis, cerebral palsy,

TABLE 8-3

Myelodysplasia—14 Cases

Combined with anterior procedure—13
    1 myelodysplasia had posterior only, idiopathic-type curve in thoracic area with myelodysplasia
      at L5 and S1
    3 Zielke
    7 multiple diskectomies
Posterior procedures—5
    3 myelodysplasia resections
    1 vertebrectomy
    1 osteotomy
Braced—6
    5 crutch-type spine brace
    1 Kosair Scoliosis Orthosis
Not braced—8
Estimated blood loss—1193 cc/case
Percentage of correction
    58.50%—scoliosis
    48.40%—kyphosis
Operating time
    5.20 hours—per case
Complications—8
    Dural leaks—cleared up with bed rest
    Wound infection—staph with prominent wires
                    —staph with migrating prominent rod
    Wound breakdown over area of myeloplastic skin
    Cardiopulmonary arrest—successful resuscitation
    Bronchial plug—bronchoscope
    Brace pressure sore
    Hematuria—questionable etiology
Percentage of complications—57%

TABLE 8-4

Muscular Dystrophy—5 Cases

Combined with anterior procedure—1
    1 with halo traction and Zielke
Braced—1
    1 crutch-type spine brace
Not braced—4
Estimated blood loss—1500 cc/case
Percentage of correction—47%
Operating time
    5.53 hours—per case
Complications—1
    1 pulmonary arrest, death, 48 hours after surgery
Percentage of complications—20%

TABLE 8-5

Tumor—6 Cases

---

1 active metastatic
1 active exostosia
2 ependymoma—kyphosis after excision with paraplegia (previous surgery)
1 astrocytoma—kyphoscoliosis status after incomplete excision in August 1978 with radiation
1 active osteoblastoma
Combined with anterior procedure—4
    2 multiple diskectomies
    1 ependymoma debulking tumor
    1 vertebrectomy
Braced—5
Not braced—1
Estimated blood loss—1258.30 cc/case
Operating time
    5.10 hours—per case
Complications—2
    1 brace pressure care
    1 staph infection area—wound breakdown
Percentage of complications—33.30%

TABLE 8-6

Cerebral Palsy/Head Injuries—27 Cases

Combined with anterior procedure—10
    6 Zielke
    1 diskectomy and vertebrectomy
    3 multiple diskectomies
Braced—4
Not braced—23
Estimated blood loss—1617.50 cc/case
Operating time
    4.91 hours—per case
Complications—9
    Infection—deep strep, deep staph, bone graft donor site
    Wound dehiscence
    Prominent rods requiring shortening
    Rods too short with wires slipped
    Kyphosis above fusion—fusion too short
Percentage of complications—33.30%

---

myelodysplasia, tumors, late posttraumatic kyphosis, progressive kyphosis secondary to osteoporosis associated with pain, and kyphoscoliosis secondary to poliomyelitis. Of these patients, 29 underwent both anterior and posterior procedures.

TABLE 8-7

Trauma—27 Cases

---

20 acute fractures
      8 with neurologic deficit
7 old fractures
      1 with neurologic deficit
Combined with anterior procedure—13
   10 vertebrectomies
      9 acute
      1 old
   3 diskectomies
      1 old after laminectomy
      2 multiple compression fractures T8 to T11
Estimated blood loss—200 cc to 4000 cc
   996.00 cc—per case
Operating time
   3.97 hours—per case
Braced—17
Not braced—7
   3 other
Complications—9
   Thrombophlebitis
   Collapse of fracture site—increased leg pain
                             no kyphosis
   Hemothorax—after rodding
   Wound dehiscence
   Prominent wire—1 requiring removal
                 —1 not removed
   Wound hematoma
Percentage of complications—33.30%
Neurologic return was rewarding

All patients undergoing two-stage procedures were braced postoperatively. Patients who had received a lumbar fusion, particularly lumbosacral fusions, were braced, since a significant percentage of these types of patients suffered wire breakage in our earlier study. The clinical significance of this is not known at the present time, however. The remainder of the patients were braced based upon the following factors: severe kyphosis present prior to surgery or persistent kyphosis following surgery, severe osteopenia, or muscle imbalance (such as in patients with dysplasia and cerebral palsy).

The complication rate in the second group of patients has been much lower, although the length of follow-up is shorter. However, as in the first group, most complications presented in the first six months. Of the 221 patients in Part II, there have been no deaths. Two deep wound infections have occurred. One was in a patient with myelodysplasia associated with wound dehiscence, and the other was in a patient who had a lumbar fusion for degenerative spondylosis of the lumbar spine. Two nonunions have occurred. One wire breakage without rod failure or loss of correction was noted.

TABLE 8-8

Spondylolisthesis—15 Cases

---

3 redo
Combined with neurologic procedure—4
Combined with anterior procedure—2
Braced—3
Not braced—7
    3 other—partial bracing with no sitting
Estimated blood loss—1285.70 cc/case
Operating time
    3.65 hours—per case
Complications—3
    Broken wires
    Vocal cord paralysis
    Transient S1 and S2 sensory loss with neurologic bladder—persistent
Percentage of complications—20%

TABLE 8-9

Polio—2 Cases

Combined with anterior procedure—2
    1 Zielke
    1 discectomy
Braced—1
    1 Kosair Scoliosis Orthosis
Not braced—1
Estimated blood loss—1650 cc
Operating time
    5.00 hours—per case
Percentage of correction
    33%—scoliosis
    67%—kyphosis
Complications—0
Percentage of complications—0

TABLE 8-10

Ankylosing Spondylitis—1 Case

---

1 salvage procedure status after osteotomy and intraoperative paraplegia (recovered)
No brace
Estimated blood loss—700 cc
Operating time—3.50 hours

TABLE 8-11

Neurofibromatosis—3 Cases

Combined with anterior procedure—2
Braced—1
Not braced—1
Estimated blood loss—1021 cc/case
Operating time
     4.42 hours—per case
Complications—0
Percentage of complications—0

TABLE 8-12

Scheuermann's Kyphosis—4 Cases

Combined with anterior procedure—4
     4 multiple diskectomies
Estimated blood loss—1500 cc/case
Operating time
     5.75 hours—per case
Braced—2
Not braced—1
     Other—1
Complications
     Sponge left in wound
     Right lower extremity hyperesthesia and weakness—resolved

TABLE 8-13

Degenerative—4 Cases

     No anterior
Estimated blood loss—1250 cc/case

When segmental spinal instrumentation was first introduced by Dr. Eduardo Luque in the late 1970s, the double Luque rod system offered the spine surgeon a better means of correcting spinal deformities by using a stronger force segmentally distributed over the chosen area. Suddenly, the most fearful deformities could be treated; however, there were many pitfalls. With the use of double Luque instru-

TABLE 8-14

Down's Syndrome—1 Case

No anterior
Estimated blood loss—2500 cc/case
Complications
    Death

mentation, migration of the wires and, therefore, possible rotation of the L-shaped rods were distinct possibilities (Figs. 8-1 and 8-2). As the rods would rotate, the tip of the rods would then become prominent underneath the skin, giving rise to a painful bursal sac. Because the spinal canal is violated, the risk of neurologic compromise has also been greatly increased with this form of spinal instrumentation. On the other hand, greater correction can be obtained.

At the time that segmental spinal instrumentation was first introduced, it was believed that the system was so strong and offered such large corrective forces that often an anterior arthrodesis of the spine could be avoided. We have since learned that this is not the case and that anterior spinal arthrodesis continues to be indicated with this system (Figs. 8-3 and 8-4).

We still prefer to do anterior and posterior spinal fusions on paralytic collapsing spines. However, we rarely use instrumentation anteriorly for the collapsing spine. In previous years, Dwyer instrumentation was a standard procedure when combined with a posterior Harrington rod instrumentation and fusion for the paralytic deformity (Figs. 8-5 and 8-6).

Luque instrumentation has been particularly rewarding in trauma. Lordosis as well as kyphosis can usually be maintained in paraplegics. This helps to reduce the decubitus ulcers that these patients often develop over areas such as the ischial tuberosity. By maintaining the normal thoracic kyphosis as well as the normal lumbar lordosis, weight can be better distributed over the posterior aspect of the thighs as well as the buttocks, thereby preventing sores over the bony prominences such as the ischial tuberosities. In early cases, when SSI was not combined with an anterior procedure for a deficiency in the anterior spinal column, late collapse invariably occurred. Now an anterior arthrodesis is always utilized in fracture cases when it is deemed necessary. It is felt that when a severe comminuted fracture of the vertebral body exists, with greater than 50% collapse of the vertebral body and an angular deformity involving the vertebral body between T8 and L3, an anterior arthrodesis in conjunction with segmental spinal instrumentation and fusion should be seriously considered. Anterior stabilization is also necessary after extensive laminectomies have been performed (Figs. 8-7 to 8-9).

In order to guard against rod migration as well as rotation, molding of a square-shaped rod instead of two double-L rods is now preferred. This can be obtained by bending a 100-cm L-shaped rod into a rectangular configuration or by

There were 16 uncategorized cases. Table 8-15 is a summary of complications encountered.

TABLE 8-15

Complications of SSI

CARDIOPULMONARY—6 CASES
   6 cases—44%
   2 deaths—1.47%
   1 CP—0.073%
      intraoperative anesthetic—successful resuscitation
   1 thrombophlebitis
   1 hemothorax
   1 bronchial plug

NEUROLOGIC—5 CASES
   5 cases—3.67%
   1 paraplegia—with early spotty recovery—75% return to normal later
   2 limb hyperesthesia and weakness, resolved
   1 limb hyperesthesia and weakness, resolved, with persistent neurogenic bladder
   1 vocal cord paralysis—endotracheal tube

DURAL LEAK—2 CASES
   2 myelodysplasia

INFECTION—7 CASES
   7 cases—5.14%
   1 donor site staph A
   1 deep strep
   1 deep staph A
   1 superficial staph A

WOUND HEALING—5 CASES
   5 cases—3.67%
   3 dehiscence
   1 hematoma
   1 skin breakdown at myelodysplasia region

INSTRUMENT FAILURE—11 CASES
   11 cases—8.00%
      —5.14% not counting collapsed fracture
   3 fractured wires
   1 fractured ¼" rod
   1 problem wire requiring removal
   2 problem wires requiring shortening
   4 collapsed at fracture site
      3 into kyphosis
      1 kyphosis with increased leg pain

JUDGMENT ERROR—3 CASES
   1 rods too short—wires slipped off twice
   1 kyphosis above fusion mass—too short
   1 sponge left in wound

BRACE PRESSURE SORE—2 CASES
   2 cases—1.47%

HEMATOMA—1 CASE
   Unknown etiology

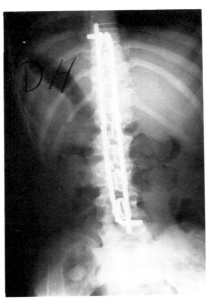
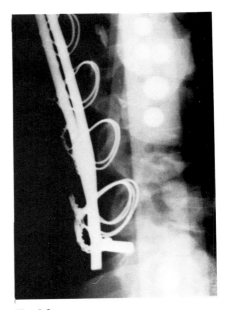

Figs. 8-1 and 8-2. The L-shaped portion of the rod is migrating, and the tip of the L-portion is pointing toward the spinal canal.

Fig. 8-2.

purchasing prebent square-shaped rods. It is felt that by placing the ends of the rectangular rod next to the adjacent spinous processes, this can help to transmit some of the axial forces across the spine, thereby preventing collapse of an L-shaped rod because of poor resistance to axial compression (Figs. 8-10 and 8-11).

Although traction is obtained with segmental spinal instrumentation simply by straightening the spine without removing any of the integrated parts, we have felt that when traction is more strongly needed, it can best be obtained with a Harrington rod instrumentation and fusion. However, segmental spinal instrumentation is certainly a stronger procedure. Thus, when correcting idiopathic scoliosis, Harrington rod instrumentation provides the desired distraction, and sublaminar wires add to the strength of the system. By using Bobechko hooks, new resistance is afforded against the upper distraction hook cutting from underneath the lamina. Also, using a Leatherman hook below adds to the stability of the system. Because we leave only one ratchet below the lower hook space, rod breakage has not been a problem in our series (Figs. 8-12 and 8-13).

A Luque system alone has not been as effective in correcting idiopathic scoliotic curves or rib humps.

Since bracing is now being used in selected cases, wire breakage has not been a problem. Although bracing is important, many times knowing how far to fuse is just as critical. Figures 8-14 and 8-15 demonstrate this point in a patient with myelodysplasia. We have since begun fusing all paralytic spines from C7 or T1 to the sacrum. These patients have very poor muscular control, and simply fusing the

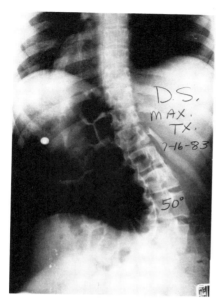 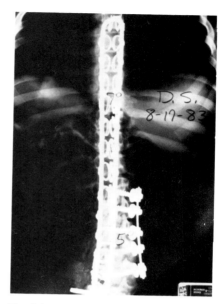

Figs. 8-3 and 8-4. An unstable spine requiring both anterior and posterior stabilization.

Fig. 8-4.

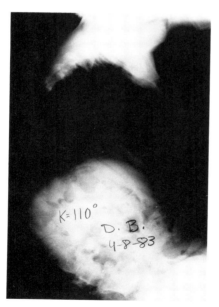 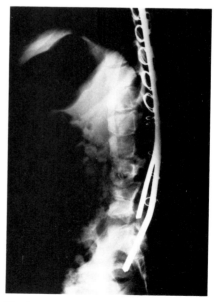

Figs. 8-5 and 8-6. A collapsing kyphotic spine requiring anterior strut graft with interbody fusion and posterior instrumentation.

Fig. 8-6.

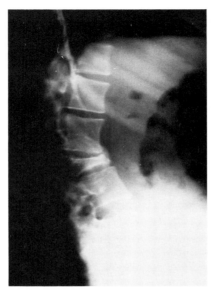

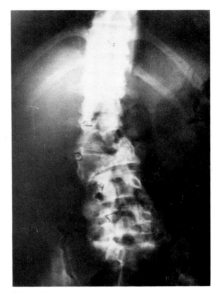

Figs. 8-7, 8-8, and 8-9. Multiple fractures, anterior arthrodesis, and posterior stabilization.

Fig. 8-8.

Fig. 8-9.

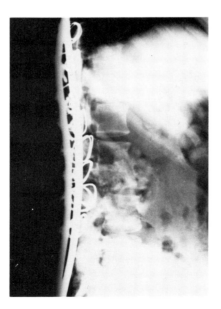

spine from the midthoracic area to the pelvis is not enough. Collapsing spines should be fused from the lower cervical vertebrae or at least from T1 to the sacrum.

Segmental spinal instrumentation and fusion is an effective modality for correction of a multitude of spinal deformities. Many pitfalls are present. Careful

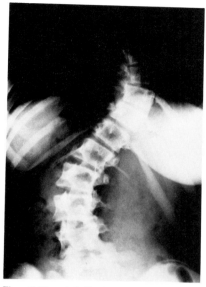
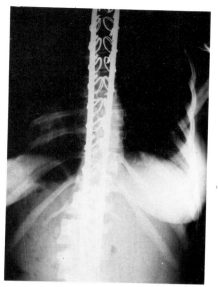

Figs. 8-10 and 8-11. An idiopathic scoliosis with Luque loop or rectangular rod to prevent collapse.

Fig. 8-11.

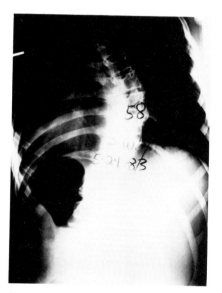
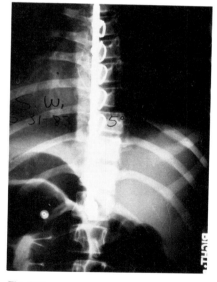

Figs. 8-12 and 8-13. An idiopathic scoliosis using a Harrington rod, two upper hooks (Bobechko), one lower hook (Leatherman), and segmental wires (Luque).

Fig. 8-13.

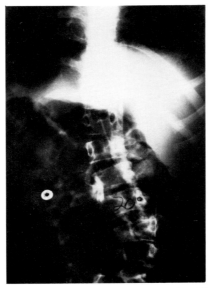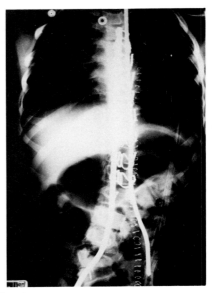

Figs. 8-14 and 8-15. A myelodysplasia fused from T3 to the sacrum.

attention to detail in planning as well as technical expertise is a must. As in any spinal instrumentation, this system must be combined with a good fusion mass. This instrumentation, like any other, is doomed to failure when combined with a poor fusion mass.

Summary

There is no question that the SSI system is well established and will play an important role in the treatment of unstable spines. This system gives greater stability and has additional corrective forces that are not available with other systems.

It is a mode of spinal surgery that needs to be integrated with existing experience. As in other types of instrumentation, one must devise the treatment plan to fit the patient's needs and not alter the patient's needs to fit the surgeon's operation.

As we have seen from the history of spinal surgery, those techniques that have been combined with poor fusions have been doomed to failure. Any time we deal with a new system or operative procedure, the prognosis is guarded if we deviate from tried and proven principles. With correction of deformity after a well-executed

SSI procedure and a solid fusion mass, along with good management of the patient, however, the prognosis is excellent.

Editor's Commentary

In this group of 357 SSI cases reported by Leatherman et al, there are several important considerations to be discussed. The most important aspect is the high incidence of complications in the first group of patients. There were a total of 42 problems in 141 cases (30%), some of them very grave, including death, paraplegia, and nerve root damage. The type of patient and the duration of some of these operations certainly account for many of these complications. In other series, a much lower rate of complications has been reported.[2,5-9] The number of complications in this first series of patients directly attributable to SSI is 11, or 8%, and three of them my coauthors consider judgment error. No specific numbers are given in their second series of 216 patients, and no degrees of pathology and correction.

Their indications for SSI are broader in their second series. Their limitations also are broader; they feel that internal distraction seems to be an ultimate necessity, and they advocate Harrington rods, Bobechko hooks, and Leatherman hooks to make the instrumentation "safer." They also advocate the use of bracing in selected cases. There is frequent use of anterior and posterior surgery, in essence shortening procedures. In the authors' opinion, SSI has not been effective in correcting idiopathic scoliosis or the rib hump.

At this time, the treatment of idiopathic scoliosis with SSI is a controversial subject. There are those who feel that there is no place for SSI in idiopathic scoliosis (Leatherman, Leiponis, Bunch, and Longstein).[1,3,4] There are others who feel that it attains a correction at least equal to that of other types of instrumentation and gives added advantages—better fixation without increasing the risk or complication rate.[2,5-9] In my personal experience, I have gone through a learning curve. In my first group of patients, 58% correction was achieved with Harri-Luques. At first, this reflected good preoperative correction, but the last 11° were without external support. The incidence of complications in this group of patients was 29%; 17% were transient neurologic complications. The average follow-up in this group of idiopathic patients is eight years. There was one pseudarthrosis.

In the second group of 13 patients with idiopathic scoliosis, with an average follow-up of 7½ years, more surgery was done. They received Harrington rods with sublaminar wiring or a straight rod on the convex side, or both. The correction was correspondingly better—72% (four patients in this group had primary anterior procedures). Still the complication rate was high (22%), and the loss of correction without external fixation postoperatively was 16°. The end result remained equal to that of group one, ± 50% correction.

The third group of patients with idiopathic scoliosis involved 24 individuals. Average follow-up was six years and three months. As in groups one and two, three-fourths were females and only one-fourth were males. The average deformity (Cobb) was 67° and the average age was 16 years in all three groups.

In group three, the spines were balanced with three-dimensional molded L rods, and compensatory curves were created. A 63% correction was obtained in the AP aspect, and for the first time, normal sagittal curves were either kept or produced. The average loss of correction was 6° owing to one thoracolumbar pseudarthrosis. There was one neurologic complication that resolved satisfactorily without removal of the instrumentation.

Group four includes 14 patients with only a four-year, two-month follow-up. Six had a double procedure. The average deformity was 73%, the average correction 64%. Less force was used in instrumenting the spine. There was only a 1° average loss of correction at follow-up. No complications were encountered. Two patients used postoperative immobilization.

The final group of 42 patients has an average follow-up of one year and eight months. As in all other groups, we included no growing children or curves over 90°. The average deformity in this group was 75°, and average correction was 69%. Thirteen patients had double procedures. The average loss of correction was 2°. There were no complications. Four of these patients used postoperative casting; all others were only prohibited from contact sports.

As can easily be seen, as time has gone on, more anterior surgery, more destruction of the deformity, and more balancing of residual curves have resulted in fewer complications and better final corrections. It is only fair to say that in the fifth group, 17 patients received closed-loop SSI to prevent loss of correction.

There is no doubt that using a cast or brace postoperatively might be relatively important in New York, but it can be very significant in tropical weather. Again, SSI must be tailored to the orthopedic center, to the orthopedist, and principally to the patient and his deformity.

SSI has focused attention on several anatomic and clinical facts that have been evident to spine surgeons for many years, yet nothing has been done about them. *These are not a formula for correcting spine deformity.* Some of these principles are:

1. *The spine is an anatomic segmented structure!*
2. The spine has a three-dimensional configuration physiologically and anatomically. Sagittal curves are normal and must be preserved.
3. In the axial plane, the spine is also segmental and three-dimensional (and to my knowledge, no existing procedure has adequately resolved this deformity).
4. In the thoracic segments, this axial segmental plane is a ring that comprises (in 10 levels) the sternum, the ribs, and the corresponding vertebrae, each with two attachments on either side.
5. Spinal deformity is segmental and must be dealt with in that way. For example, there may be a deformity of the end vertebrae in scoliosis, and consequently the

biomechanics are not the same as those at the apex. The mechanical forces involved in spondylolisthesis are different at the site of the deformity than at adjacent levels that are part of a normal sagittal curve. The pathology and biomechanics of a degenerative spine are entirely different at a level with anterior compression (eg, disk protrusion), a degenerative rotational spondylolisthesis, a hypertrophic osteoarthritic facet, a hyperplastic yellow ligament, or a neurologic complication of unmentionable possibilities. All these examples of the segmentalization of spinal pathology do not take into consideration anything about individualization according to the patient's particular pathology, way of life, prognosis, and socio-psychomotor necessities and adaptation.

6. All corrections of the spine include lengthening. (A very careful distinction has to be made between increase in height and actual lengthening of vertebral and paravertebral structures.)

7. Most corrections of spinal pathology are done using the middle column (Denis) as a fulcrum, but it is also true that all soft tissues migrate to the concave side of the deformity. Consequently, all bony corrections will correspond directly with an elongation of soft tissues by an arc described from the center of rotation to the position of structural deformity of the soft tissue structures in question. This means vascular, neurologic, muscular, ligamentous, or other structures.

This obviously will be true in the correction of the axial plane and apical rotation, or in the correction of collapsing scoliosis in the elderly patient with a calcified aorta. Scoliotic kyphotic or spondylolisthesic deformities are other examples.

8. All forces of correction have been put at the disposal of the spine surgeon. Distraction is not excluded but is balanced with lateral bend, pressure over the apex, torque moments, lateral traction, posterior traction, and the use of lever arms. At some point, at an individual or segmental level, any of these forces or combination thereof may become dangerous or nullify each other.

9. The spine, lying in the midline of the body and being a segmental structure, needs: (1) bilateral immobilization, (2) segmental immobilization, (3) if totally unstable, anterior and posterior immobilization.

10. With our present techniques, some deformities (due to their intrinsic pathology) are corrected with less danger by shortening procedures (laminotomy, laminectomy, diskectomy, corpectomy, vertebrectomy, and so forth) than by distraction (which is achieved with simple bony correction or added forces).

11. Some deformities or particular patients should not necessarily be corrected or should be corrected in a limited fashion. Our goal is anatomic and physiologic balance, avoiding complications.

12. In growing children, instrumentation not only has led us to retain early treatment of spinal pathology but is also being considered in the prevention of developing deformity.

13. Probably the most important realization in the first decade of SSI use has been that the main objective in spine surgery is not correction of the deformity, better prognosis for life expectancy, or even better immediate comfort, but a better way of life, as long as it lasts.

Obviously, our options are many, ever changing, and improving all the time. We can choose between surgery vs. conservative therapy, lengthening vs. shortening procedures, rigid internal fixation vs. external immobilization, and so forth. In the end, however, success or failure will depend on our personal understanding as physicians of the necessities of our patients, on our knowledge and judgment as individuals, and ultimately on our technical expertise. To do the right procedure for each particular patient in his particular environment is our goal.

References

1. Bunch HW, Chapman GR: Patient preferences in scoliosis surgery. Paper presented at 18th annual meeting, Scoliosis Research Society, New Orleans, LA, 1983.
2. Kahn A, Frank DJ, Shank M: Sublaminar wiring in S.S.I. Paper presented at 18th annual meeting, Scoliosis Research Society, New Orleans, LA, 1983.
3. Leiponis JF, Bunch HW, Lorser E, Daley M, Gogan WJ: Spinal cord injury during segmental sublaminar spinal instrumentation. An animal model. Paper presented at 18th annual meeting, Scoliosis Research Society, New Orleans, LA, 1983.
4. Lonstein J: Spinal Deformities Course. Bal Harbour, Florida, November 1983.
5. Odom J, Brown CW, Donaldson DH: Spinal deformity corrections with combination Harrington rods and Luque rods/wires. Paper presented at 18th annual meeting, Scoliosis Research Society, New Orleans, LA, 1983.
6. Rinsky LA, Kane N, Bleck E, Gamble J, Stanford VK: Treatment of idiopathic scoliosis with SSI. Preliminary results. Paper presented at 18th annual meeting, Scoliosis Research Society, New Orleans, LA, 1983.
7. Shufflebarger HL, Price CT, Riddick M: L-rod instrumentation and spinal fusion: The Florida experience. Paper presented at 18th annual meeting, Scoliosis Research Society, New Orleans, LA, 1983.
8. Sussman M: Advantage of early stabilization fusion of scoliosis patients with Duchenne muscular dystrophy. Paper presented at 18th annual meeting, Scoliosis Research Society, New Orleans, LA, 1983.
9. Taddonio RH, Weller K, Appel M: A comparison of patients with idiopathic scoliosis managed with and without post-operative immobilization following segmental spinal instrumentation with Luque rods: A preliminary report. Paper presented at 18th annual meeting, Scoliosis Research Society, New Orleans, LA, 1983.

Basic Considerations
in Pelvic Fixation Cases

9

Introduction and Indications

UNTIL THE PRESENT L-ROD TECHNIQUES of pelvic fixation became available, the decision to extend surgical instrumentation and spinal arthrodesis to the pelvis implied major morbidity for the patient.[2,3,6] Prolonged recumbency, a body cast that encased at least one thigh, loss of lumbar lordosis, and a high risk of pseudarthrosis were enough to dampen anyone's enthusiasm for lumbosacral fusion.[13] Even against that backdrop, the risk-gain factor for some individuals made fusion to the pelvis the best available option.[8,10,14,19-21,23,24] No other measure controls the deformity in a person with neuromuscular scoliosis associated with fixed pelvic obliquity. The adult with back pain secondary to a curve extending into the lumbosacral spine with significant degenerative changes has a problem best solved by fusion into the pelvis. When scoliosis of operative severity is associated with an oblique lumbosacral junction, fusion must extend to the pelvis if the optimum result is to be realized. Presently, with effective techniques

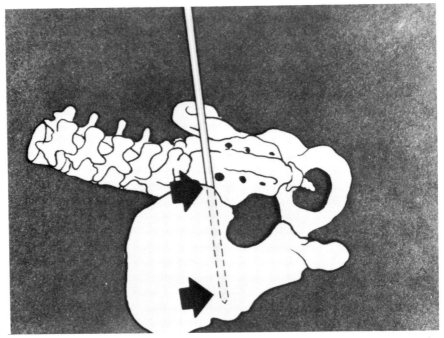

Fig. 9-1. The Galveston technique of pelvic fixation involves driving a Steinmann pin across the posterior column of the ilium into the transverse bar as shown in *A* to establish a track and subsequently driving a portion of the L-rod implant along the established track as shown in *B* to provide pelvic fixation. *C,* a photograph of an anatomic specimen with implanted pelvic fixation shows ideal placement. A window has been cut in the lateral ilium so that the intraosseous portion of the implant may be seen. (Reproduced with permission: Bobit Publishing, Contemporary Orthopaedics 7(3):51-61, 1983.)

for pelvic immobilization and fusion, we feel that anyone requiring instrumentation to the fifth lumbar vertebra would best be treated by arthrodesis to the pelvis, since there is emerging evidence of long-term problems with fusions that end at L4 or L5.

Presently, considerable variation in surgical strategy, surgical technique, and use of materials may be seen from one institution to another in its approach to the scoliosis patient needing pelvic fixation. Figure 9-1 shows the basic geometry of the Galveston technique. Our approach has been an evolutionary one focused on the most effective method for managing these patients, L-rod instrumentation.[4-6] Herein we discuss the more important factors to be considered in the pelvic fixation patient, present the Galveston technique of pelvic fixation, comment on some of the incompletely defined and controversial variables, and list the more common errors to be avoided.

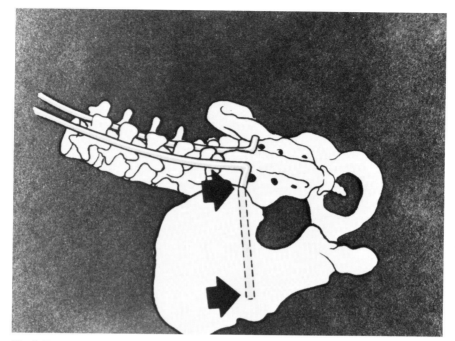

Fig. 9-1*B*.

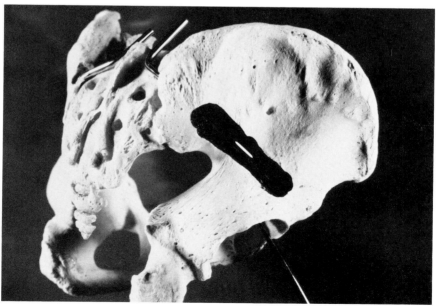

Fig. 9-1*C*.

Alignment

The provision of precise compensation, good truncal balance, and balanced secondary spinal contours is of critical importance in the patient undergoing pelvic fixation.[6,12] Because of the nature of the diseases that underlie scoliosis needing fusion to the sacrum, the most frequent instrumentation extends from the second or third thoracic vertebra to the pelvis. Failure to achieve compensation and truncal balance yields an uneven sitting base, which is a problem—a very serious one for the individual with insensitive skin over the buttocks. Loss of lumbar lordosis—hypolordosis, a generally recognized complication of distraction instrumentation—can also be a problem with Luque rod instrumentation (LRI) to the pelvis when the rods are not properly shaped. With long instrumentations, balanced thoracic kyphosis and lumbar lordosis are essential. Relatively more thoracic kyphosis than lumbar lordosis produces a flexed trunk posture, which resembles in secondary consequences the hypolordosis, flat back syndrome, or jump position seen with Harrington instrumentation. The combination of too much lumbar lordosis and too little thoracic kyphosis causes an extended trunk posture, which can be a very serious problem for the patient with limited hip flexion.[12]

Careful planning and preparation for the LRI to the pelvis is key to achieving spinal alignment. Initially, a radiographic estimate of curve flexibility should be made. Bending films are insufficient in all but the earliest mild scoliosis seen in neuromuscular disease such as muscular dystrophy or spinal muscular atrophy. Only stretch films can demonstrate exactly what will be needed to effect the best possible truncal balance and compensation. Most commonly, there will be a need to introduce a compensatory curve. Occasionally, when there is a double curve, one curve will be more flexible than the other. In such an instance, maximum correction of both curves could result in severe decompensation. By measuring the lateral deviation and compensation on a stretch film, one will know in advance what the best possible outcome is and can plan the best means to achieve it. To begin an LRI to the pelvis without a definite plan invites a compromised outcome.

In some cases, the major curve will be so severe that acceptable correction is initially not possible. We perform an anterior release and fusion over the extent of the major curve when improved correctability would enhance the surgical result.[12] In such a case, the anterior release and fusion constitutes the first operation in a two-stage correction. Following it, between stages, the patient is kept in tong gravity traction on a CircOLectric bed for about two weeks. Just prior to the second-stage LRI, a stretch film is made, and based on the "new" correctability, the LRI is planned. The anterior release and fusion is usually needed when the major deformity will not passively correct to less than 50 degrees, when there is no other way to effect compensation, and when circumferential arthrodesis is needed. With the exception of myelomeningocele scoliosis in the region of vertebral arch deficiency, acceptably correctable neuromuscular scoliosis can be effectively managed with single-stage LRI and fusion.[2,3] Whereas anterior arthrodesis greatly

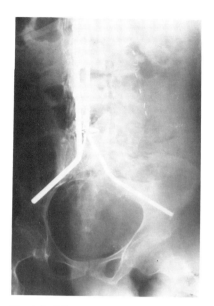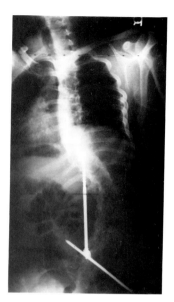

Fig. 9-2. This relatively large 24-year-old man, who had poliomyelitis as a child, is shown as an example of pelvic fixation because his circumstance illustrates many of the less straightforward points to be considered. Although he has flailed lower extremities and is nonambulatory, he is an accomplished wheelchair athlete. *A*, His pelvic fixation in situ. Note the asymmetry of the pelvis, necessitating spinal alignment with reference to the ischial tuberosities rather than the top of the iliac crest. Observe that because of his size, a one-fourth inch rod has been applied to one side and a 3/16-inch rod to the other. Because the posterior spinal anatomy has been distorted by a previous arthrodesis, the bends in the pelvis-fixing portions of the L-rod have been adapted to his anatomy. *B*, He presented with a severe fixed pelvic obliquity, which was secured by a successful arthrodesis in poor alignment. *C*, The first critical step was establishment of correctability. This was accomplished by anterior and posterior vertebral osteotomies and tong gravity traction. This stretch film shows the degree of correctability present just prior to L-rod instrumentation with pelvic fixation. *D*, This sitting postoperative AP view shows acceptable truncal balance and one and one-half cm decompensation to the left. *E*, The forward projection of the pelvic limbs of the implant can be seen on this postoperative lateral view. It was not possible to introduce more lordosis into the lumbar spine. The wiring technique is a revision one, with wires passing between the diploe of a mature fusion in the lumbar region and sublaminarly in the thoracic spine. *F* and *G*, 45-degree oblique pelvic outlet views show the pelvic limbs of the rods passing cleanly across the posterior columns of the ilia and into the transverse bars. *H* and *I*, Clinical photos approximately one week after L-rod instrumentation document reasonable sitting alignment on a hard horizontal surface.

improves the fusion rate with Harrington instrumentation, the anterior fusion is not critical in L-rod instrumentations.[2,3,8] When great force is required to correct and align the spine satisfactorily on a stretch film, it is best to do a two-stage correction, because even L-rods will bend under conditions of excessive loading.[6,26] In our experience with rigid neuromuscular curves averaging an 88.1° Cobb angle in severity, initial stress correction was 27.7%. Following anterior release and fusion (ARF) and traction, correction improved to 57.2%, and a slight gain to 63.8%

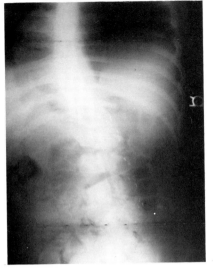

Fig. 9-2*C*.

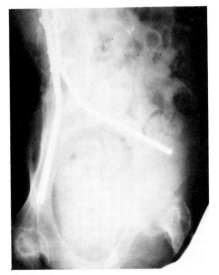

Fig. 9-2*E*.

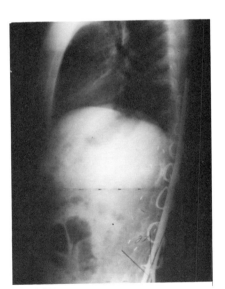

Fig. 9-2*F*.

occurred with LRI.[12] Usually, one can gain a 7° to 12° correction per motion segment with the two-stage ARF-LRI approach. These figures are statistically no different from the correction reported for two-stage anterior instrumentation followed by Harrington instrumentation.[8,10,14,19-21,23,24] Although our percentage of correction of pelvic obliquity, 67.4%, was also statistically the same as reported for two-stage corrections, we feel that much better corrections are possible with

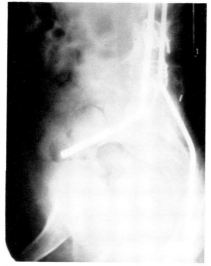

Fig. 9-2*G*.

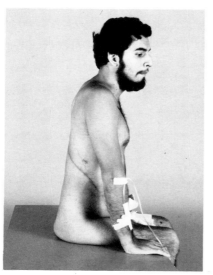

Fig. 9-2*H*

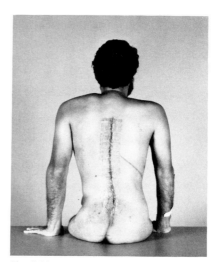

Fig. 9-2*I*.

planned LRI.[6,12] From experience with some of our early cases, we realized that better planning would have led to an improved result. The case shown in Figure 9-2 illustrates a planned solution to a moderately severe problem.

A problem that has not been emphasized in the literature is that the patient with weak trunk musculature may develop kyphosis above an area of spinal instrumentation when the instrumentation extends from the mid- or low thoracic region into the pelvis. Because of this problem, we generally extend instrumentation for our neuromuscular cases from the second or third thoracic vertebra to the pelvis.

Biomechanics

When pelvic fixation is done in conjunction with instrumentation for scoliosis, the long spinal segment that has undergone instrumentation above the pelvis acts as a lever, concentrating lateral bending, flexion-extension, and torsional stresses at the lumbopelvic junction. This is a straightforward mechanical problem that can be approached from a basic consideration of moments—load equals force multiplied by distance. Since the axis for movements at the lumbosacral junction is somewhere in the L5-S1 disk, that approximate site can be used for our mechanical considerations. Ideally, one would like to increase the leverage of the pelvis-fixing implant in all directions so that all stresses could be resisted at the best mechanical advantage. Also, the levers for resisting these stresses would be as long as possible so that the load at the ends of the levers, and therefore on the tissue, would be so small that the tissue would not be strained to its yielding point.

The goals are clear, but the geometry of the human pelvis limits the available options. Because usable sites of sacral fixation lie close to the L5-S1 disk—the axis of movement—only a short lever arm is possible; therefore, any type of sacral fixation is a priori at a severe mechanical disadvantage. One could improve the mechanics of pelvic fixation by running a limb of each L-rod coronally through the posterior ilium, but because the ilia are rather thin bones that lie oblique to the coronal plane, the amount of bony tissue available for loading is very limited. Furthermore, only a few centimeters of leverage above that for sacral fixation is gained. Worst of all, because with this rod geometry the limbs of the implant used to fix the pelvis lie in the coronal plane, and flexion-extension takes place about a coronal plane axis, there is no leverage at all, which provides no advantage against flexion-extension movements. The full load will be seen as either direct compression or tension at the site of pelvic fixation.

How can any leverage for resisting flexion-extension forces be gained? Pelvic geometry limits us to one option: The limb of the pelvic portion of each of the L-rods can be bent to follow the forward, anterolateral, inclination of the ilium. Because of the oblique orientation, additional leverage for resisting lateral bending stresses will be gained as well. Once again, a constraining anatomic factor comes into play; the central area of the ilium, appropriately labeled the membranous portion, is so thin that there is no way to pass the limb of an implant through it. When pelvic limbs that have been angled forward are driven into the ilium at the level of the membranous portion, they inevitably fracture through the iliac cortex, thereby limiting the leverage that can be gained. Furthermore, in actual clinical experience, bicortical fixation, which may be suspected to have an advantage, in fact has no advantage at all.[6]

The problem of inadequate leverage, which is in essence a problem of too short a tract through the ilium, could theoretically be solved by putting the pelvic-fixing limb of the implant above or below the membranous portion of the ilium. The geometry of lower placement is much more attractive because (1) the posterior column of the ilium is much straighter than the wing of the ilium, (2) with the lower placement one gains a sacral buttressing effect, and (3) high placement would interfere with taking a posterior iliac crest bone graft. The longest levers can best be provided by driving the pelvic limb of the L-rod through the posterior column and into the transverse bar of the ilium. Such placement is as close as possible to the biomechanical ideal in pelvic fixation.

Using the mechanically ideal placement of pelvic limbs carries the psychomotor penalty of geometric complexity and the surgical penalty of extensive exposure of the posterior ilia. The theoretical is fine, but something less than ideal, if it would achieve the goals of secure pelvic fixation and a high rate of lumbopelvic arthrodesis, it might be preferable.

The only way to assess the minimal effective technique is clinical trial. In our experience, the triangular base-transverse bar technique of pelvic fixation was the only one that effectively immobilized the pelvis and produced an acceptable fusion rate without the need for a postoperative cast or brace. Fixation at the level of the membranous portion of the ilium was associated with a high incidence of pelvic loosening and a high rate of lumbosacral pseudarthroses—40%.[6] Broadstone and Leatherman, in their series of pelvic fixation cases with straight-through-the-ilium implant geometry, had a high pseudarthrosis rate, 22%, when the patients were not immobilized in a cast.[9] In the Galveston series, triangular base-transverse bar fixation yielded an overall 96% rate of successful lumbosacral arthrodesis in scoliosis cases.[6] Pelvic immobilization appeared to be best when the pelvic limb entered the ilium at the lower margin of the posterior superior iliac spine, passed within one and one-half centimeters of the sciatic notch, and penetrated a minimal depth of six centimeters. We suspect that the lower the implant placement, the greater the sacral buttressing effect at the caudal extreme of the spinal portion of the rods.

Even in experienced hands, imperfect placement of the pelvic limbs may occasionally occur. When such is the circumstance, some loss of correction and failure of lumbosacral arthrodesis are significant possibilities if the patient is left unprotected. Broadstone and Leatherman, in their series of nine cases of straight-through-the-ilium pelvic fixations, reported no pseudarthroses when the patient was placed in a postoperative cast.[9] On the basis of their experience, it seems highly advantageous to use a postoperative cast when the implants penetrate the ilium or are poorly placed, or when one is using a mechanically inferior technique. The guiding principle is that successful fusion of the portion of the spine undergoing instrumentation to the pelvis requires good immobilization.

An incompletely defined variable at the present time is the optimum stiffness of the lumbosacral end of the L-rod implant. While our techniques have been documented to be effective in neuromuscular scoliosis patients, thereby indicating adequate stiffness, a documented experience with large, neurologically normal adult patients has not been compiled. It is possible that such a group might benefit from increased implant stiffness; if so, the use of larger rods or rigid coupling devices may be a reasonable consideration.[6,26] Only further clinical experience can sort out these possibilities.

Materials

Until the summer of 1981, we used exclusively dual 3/16-inch 3/16 stainless steel rods and .048-inch (1.2 millimeter, 16 gauge) fully annealed 3/16 stainless steel wire. With these materials, we documented an 8% rate of wire breakage among the scoliosis patients during the first postsurgical year and a 10% rate of wire breakage in fracture cases, usually during the first several postoperative months. Concern over what we considered to be excessive wire failure provoked us to consider alloys with better performance-as-a-wire characteristics than stainless steel. MP-35-N was identified as a material with better fatigue properties, excellent work hardening, acceptable notch sensitivity, availability as a fully annealed wire, and Young's modulus similar to stainless steel. Titanium was found to have good fatigue properties, poor work hardening, marked notch sensitivity, availability as a fully annealed wire, and a Young's modulus roughly half that of stainless steel. MP-35-N seemed an ideal alternative to stainless steel and titanium an unacceptable one. We have used MP-35-N materials of the same dimension as the earlier stainless steel exclusively since the summer of 1981. To date, we have seen only one broken wire in a very active boy with idiopathic scoliosis.

In our review of pelvic fixation cases, we found that with the pelvic limb of the implant well secured, some bending of the spinal portion sometimes occurred.[6] This was especially likely in the individual who had athetoid cerebral palsy and had undergone instrumentation from high in the thoracic spine to the pelvis. The worst example we had was an 8° bend, which resulted in a 4½-centimeter loss of compensation. There are many possible solutions to the problem; until the best of them has been sorted out, we suggest using at least one 1/4-inch rod for instrumentation of very large individuals and those with athetoid cerebral palsy when long instrumentations with pelvic fixation are performed.

Both stainless steel and MP-35-N have the disadvantage of causing malignant transformation in rats, a phenomenon related to their nickel content.[7,17,27] No epidemiologic data are available at this time, and we cannot put the matter into perspective. Presently, we do not have non-nickel-containing alloys that could reasonably be expected to function satisfactorily with today's designs of spinal implants. Our practice is to inform our patients of our concern and ignorance, advise them that the implant can be removed when the fusion is mature, and allow them to make the decision what to do. To this time, no one has elected to have an implant removed for fear of cancer.

For the foreseeable future, we plan to keep using the MP-35-N materials because of their mechanical superiority.

Technique

The basic geometry of the Galveston triangular base-transverse bar technique is shown in Figure 9-1. When L-rod fixation to the pelvis is performed, acute bends divide the implant into three segments: one that lies intraosseously in the ilium, one that passes across the posterior surface of the sacrum, and another that runs along the length of the spinal segment that is to receive instrumentation. These regions are referred to as iliac, sacral, and spinal segments or portions.

Special instruments designed for the purpose greatly facilitate proper shaping of the pelvic end of a rod (Fig. 9-3). The sleeve benders and the pelvic rod clamp provide the leverage for making acute bends. The sleeve benders have a rounded radius at the tip of the working end to avoid scarring of the rods. The pelvic rod clamp is a modified vise grip with jaws that can grasp a rod near an acute bend. The pelvic rod guide has two parallel holes in its working end that are used to maintain the iliac portion of a rod aligned with a pelvic guide pin while the surgeon shapes the spinal portion.

Figures 9-4, 9-5, and 9-6 illustrate the text that follows. The first critical step in pelvic fixation is driving 3/16-inch in diameter Steinmann pins into the ilium along the path to be followed by the iliac portion of the rods. Wide bilateral exposure of the pelvis is necessary to do this with accuracy. Both the right and left side of the pelvis are exposed to the extent that the surgeon can hook a finger into the sciatic notch while a pelvic guide pin is driven. Visualization must be sufficient to allow accurate assessment of compensation and to permit accurate identification of the sciatic notch. The surgeon places an index finger into the sciatic notch and drives a pin intraosseously across the posterior column of the ilium. The pin enters the ilium beneath the erector spinae musculature adjacent to the posterior sacral surface. It should pass within 1.5 centimeters of the sciatic notch and penetrate a depth of at least 6 centimeters, usually 9 or 10 centimeters.

Once a pin is in place, two measurements need to be made. The first is the depth of pin penetration into the ilium. This is accomplished simply by placing another pin of the same length alongside the pelvic guide pin and measuring the difference. The second is the distance from the point of pin penetration into the ilium to the base of the sacral spinous processes. For the sake of this discussion, consider the depth of pin penetration to be ten centimeters and the distance across the posterior sacral surface to be two centimeters. When the pelvic guide pins are in

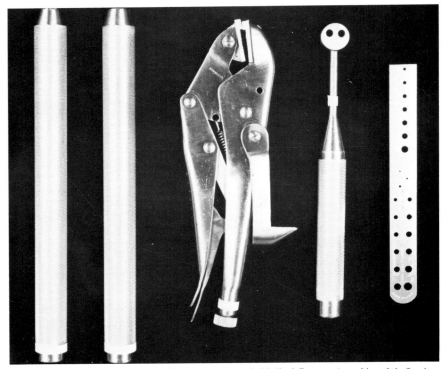

Fig. 9-3. The special instruments (available from Richards Medical Company) used in pelvic fixation include (left to right): sleeve benders, pelvic rod clamp, pelvic rod guide, and standard ruler. (Reproduced with permission: Bobit Publishing, Contemporary Orthopædics 7(3):51-61, 1983.)

position and these measurements have been made, the surgeon is ready to contour the rods.

A 60-centimeter, 3/16-inch in diameter MP-35-N rod is selected, and a sleeve bender is positioned on the rod. Grasping both the sleeve bender and rod enables one to have maximum leverage and also to control the rod and the sleeve bender without the necessity for a locking device. The combined length of the iliac and sacral segments is measured, and the sleeve bender is positioned at the point of the first bend, which will be between the spinal and sacral portions of the rod. With this length of rod protruding from the initial sleeve bender, a second sleeve bender is slipped into place, and an approximately 90-degree bend is made. Since the "L" at the top of the rod will not be used, it is cut away. This leaves a long, straight segment of rod that bends into an L, with the shorter segment representing the combined lengths of the sacral and iliac segments.

The next bend to be made is the one between the sacral and iliac segments of the rod. The two-centimeter sacral segment is measured along the short limb in the pelvic rod clamp position. Since about 1/2 centimeter in length will be gained because of the gradual radius of the bend, the tip of the clamp should lie about 1.5

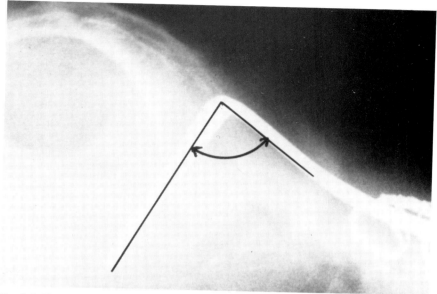

Fig. 9-4. The angle of sacral inclination is the angular relationship between the pelvic limb of the implant and the posterior surface of the sacrum. (Reproduced with permission: Bobit Publishing, Contemporary Orthopaedics 7(3):51-61, 1983.)

centimeters to provide the two-centimeter sacral segment. With the pelvic rod clamp in position, a sleeve bender is positioned on the iliac segments, and the rod is bent. The angle may vary between 45 to 65 degrees depending upon the particular case. An estimate is made by observing the angle between the pelvic guide pin and the posterior sacrum. At this point, the rod has been shaped into iliac, sacral, and spinal portions.

By looking at the previously placed Steinmann guide pins and the posterior sacrum, the angle of sacral inclination can be judged and the rods to be implanted adjusted accordingly. If adjustment is needed, the iliac portion of the rod is placed into a sleeve bender, and the angle is adjusted by making a torsional bend through the sacral segment.

At this point, shaping of the part of the implant that will afford pelvic fixation is completed, and the spinal segment must be contoured. To facilitate this, the iliac portion of the rod is positioned parallel to the appropriate guide pin by using the pelvic rod guide. The spinal segment of the rod is positioned to lie perpendicular to a line across the top of the iliac crest. A French rod bender, modified for 3/16-inch stock, is now used to place appropriate lordosis and any incomplete correction into the portion of the rod that will be affixed to the lumbar spine. Once the lumbar contour is complete, the rod is removed from the pelvic rod guide and rotated 180 degrees so that appropriate thoracic kyphosis and any incomplete thoracic correction can be bent into the implant.

The completely shaped rod to be implanted on the right side of the spine is

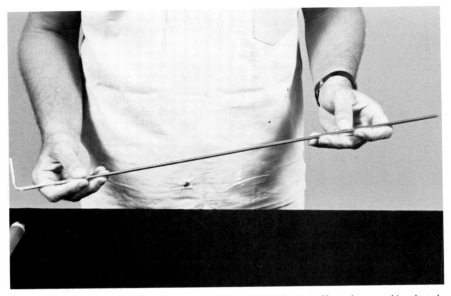

Fig. 9-5. This series of studio shots shows the rod shaping technique. *A,* 60-centimeter rod is selected from stock, and *B,* a sleeve bender is positioned on it. *C,* The combined iliac and sacral segment lengths are measured along the free end of the rod as shown. *D,* Using a second sleeve bender, an approximately 90-degree bend is made at the point that separates the spinal and sacral segments of the rod. *E,* The short limb is cut away, since it will not be used, and now one has an L-shaped rod with a long spinal segment and a shorter segment that represents the sacral and iliac portions. *F,* The length of the sacral segment is measured and the pelvic rod clamp positioned as shown. *G,* By using a combination of the pelvic rod clamp and sleeve bender, the angle between the sacral and iliac portions of the implant is made (usually it will be 55 to 60 degrees). *H,* The pelvic limb of the implant is placed in a sleeve bender, and the second sleeve bender is positioned along the spinal segment. *I,* By placing a torsional bend through the sacral segment, the angle of sacral inclination is adjusted. *J,* This picture corresponds with the operating room Figure 6*E;* while the pelvic rod guide holds the iliac segment, a French bender is used to bend appropriate lordosis into the implant. *K,* The lordosis has been completed through the lumbar region of the spinal segment. *L,* The rod is rotated 180 degrees so that the French bender can be utilized to contour appropriate thoracic kyphosis. *M,* The fully shaped rod should have balanced secondary contours. *N,* An end-on view of the pelvic end of the fully shaped rod shows the iliac, the sacral, and the beginning of the spinal segments. (Reproduced with permission: Bobit Publishing, Contemporary Orthopaedics 7(3):51-61, 1983.)

shown in Fig. 9-5*M*. Note the provision of secondary spinal contours, the angle of sacral inclination, and the previously mentioned portions of the pelvic end of the rod. The rods are inserted by extracting the pelvic guide pins and driving the iliac segment along the tract established by the guide pin. During the initial phase of driving the pelvic portion, the spinal portion should be held almost perpendicular to the patient's trunk. As it is impacted into place, it can be rotated to lie alongside the spine. The remainder of the spinal fixation is done according to usual L-rod techniques.[4]

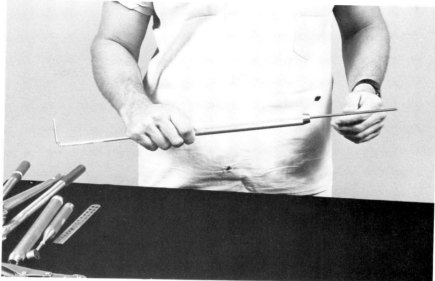

Fig. 9-5*B*.

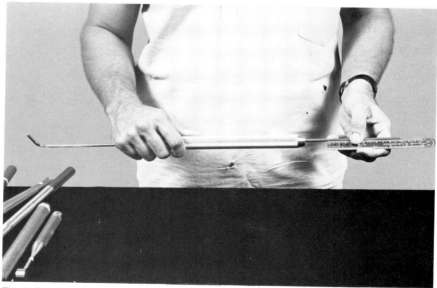

Fig. 9-5*C*.

The pathologic spinal anatomy seen in myelomeningocele patients can be accommodated with a few modifications of technique. Usually, the area of sacral rachischisis is so wide that a sacral segment of the pelvis-fixing end of a rod is not necessary; the iliac portion bends directly into the spinal portion. Just as in other

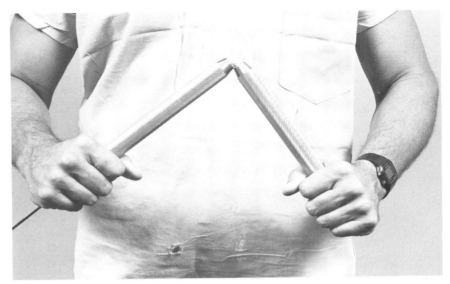

Fig. 9-5*D*

Fig. 9-5*E*.

pelvic fixation cases, a guide pin is driven along the desired track in the ilium, and the depth of penetration is measured. The long end of an L-rod is measured to this distance, and sleeve benders are used to make a sharp bend in the rod. This angle now separates the iliac and spinal segments of the rod. After recovering the short "L" and the sleeve benders, one holds the iliac segment of the rod parallel to the

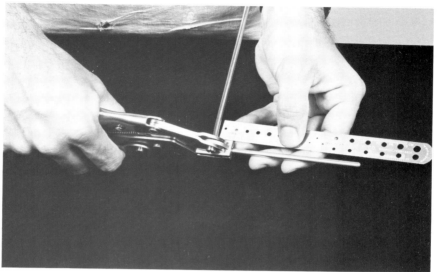

Fig. 9-5*F.*

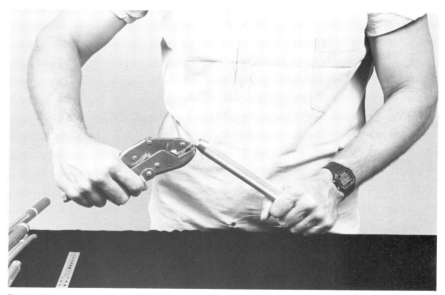

Fig. 9-5*G.*

pelvic guide pin with a pelvic rod guide and estimates the angle of bend needed to both accommodate the angle of sacral inclination and direct the spinal segment in the desired direction. Once the proper angle has been bent into the rod, the spinal segment is contoured to the desired shape. Implantation is done with the technique adapted for myelomeningocele patients.[4]

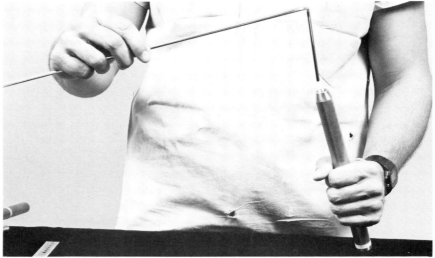

Fig. 9-5*H*.

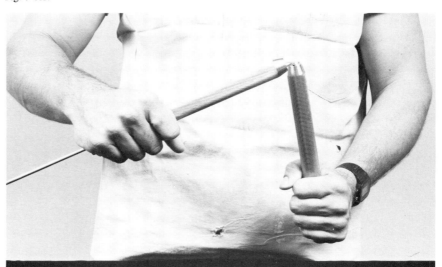

Fig. 9-5*I*.

Evaluation

Unfortunately, there has been no standard method for assessing the options for pelvic fixation. Some, such as the sacral alar hook and the sacral alar bar designed for use with the Harrington system, require such a rigorous postsurgical program

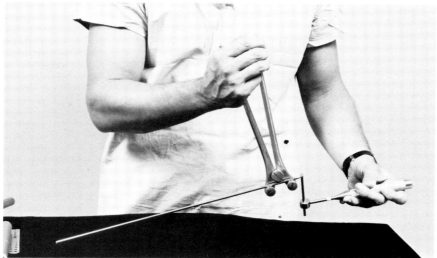

Fig. 9-5*J*.

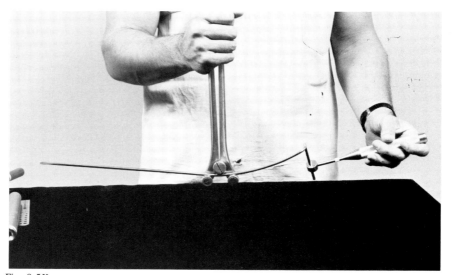

Fig. 9-5*K*.

of recumbency and exoskeletal immobilization that there seems little justification to continue their use.[16] A critical analysis of their performance as corrective devices has yet to be compiled.

In any pelvic fixation case, there are certain questions fundamental to the evaluation of implant performance. Does the implant change in position relative to the pelvis? Does the implant permit angular change to occur at the lumbosacral junction? Is there evidence of implant movement in the pelvis? Does the implant

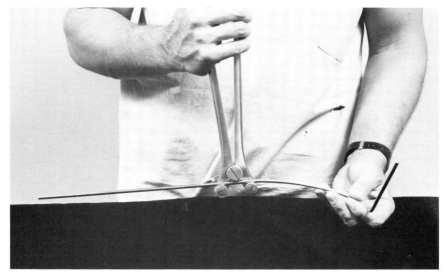

Fig. 9-5*L*.

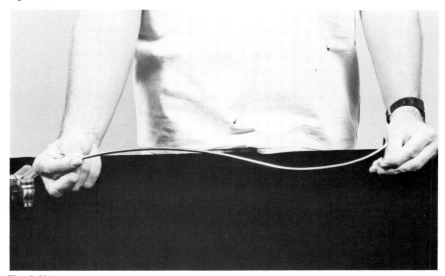

Fig. 9-5*M*.

facilitate an acceptable rate of lumbosacral fusion? Is the implant made of a material well suited for its application?

We have suggested a means of documenting the answers to these questions by a series of x-ray measurements made on a standard anteroposterior view.[6] It needs to be emphasized that for accurate measurements around the pelvis, it is critical that exactly the same landmarks be selected from x-ray film to film. A fine marking tool should be used rather than a grease pencil because the line of the latter is so

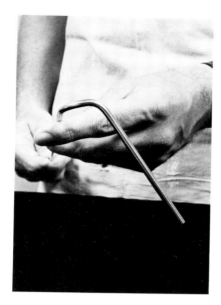

Fig. 9-5O.

broad that it introduces a small random error. Also, it is important that x-rays made at different intervals be taken with a similar technique, with the patient in the same position for each exposure. We use the standard scoliosis technique: long cassette, six-foot tube-to-film distance, centering at the level of the xyphoid, standing anteroposterior and lateral films for ambulatory patients. For nonambulatory patients, sitting films made in similar manner are taken.

Changes in the angular relationship of L4-L5 to the pelvis can be documented by the method shown in Figure 9-7A; the angle is conveniently notated—angle L4, L5-P. Changes in the relationship of the implant to the pelvis are judged by the angle between the implant and the pelvis as shown in Figure 9-7B; this value is angle I,P. A rough estimate of the movement of the pelvic limbs of the implanted rods within the ilium can be made by measuring the width of the radiolucent interval between an edge of the pelvic limb of the rod and the radiodense reactive bone that forms around it, the so-called "wiper effect." Fusion is present when homogenous, trabecular bone can be seen extending from the lateral gutters of the lumbar spine onto the sacrum. When we used these measurements to document the performance of the pelvic fixation geometries we had used, we obtained the results shown in Figure 9-7C. The best performance was seen when the pelvic limb of the rods was placed low on the ilium. It lay intraosseously through at least a six-centimeter path across the posterior column into the transverse bar of the ilium, and passed within one and one-half centimeters of the sciatic notch.

In addition to the preceding x-ray studies, we obtain 45-degree oblique pelvic outlet views preoperatively when there is any reason to suspect pelvic asymmetry, and postoperatively as a matter of routine in the postsurgical pelvic fixation

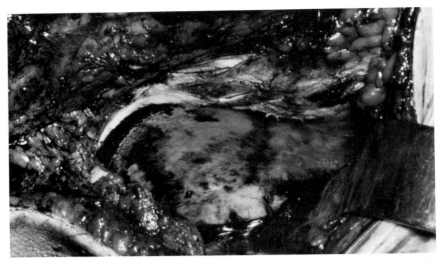

Fig. 9-6. These figures highlight some of the technical points in the operating room. *A,* The posterior ilium is exposed widely from the single midline incision. *B,* By placing a finger into the sciatic notch and positioning the pin beneath the erector spinae musculature at the inferior margin of the posterior superior iliac spine, the surgeon can aim it across the posterior column toward the transverse bar. *C,* Usually it is best for the surgeon to maintain a fix on the pelvic anatomy with one hand and maintain direction of the pin with the other; an assistant drives the pin with a mallet. *D,* Both pelvic guide pins have now been inserted. The extent of posterior pelvic visualization can be seen. *E,* Once the pelvic end of an L-rod has been shaped, the iliac portion is held parallel to a guide pin by the pelvic rod guide. *F,* With the rod thus held in an appropriate relationship to the pelvis, lordosis is bent into the portion that will attach to the lumbar spine. *G,* The point of transition from lumbar lordosis to thoracic kyphosis is identified; the rod will now be removed, rotated 180 degrees and contoured to thoracic kyphosis as shown in Figure 9-5*L.* (Reproduced with permission: Bobit Publishing, Contemporary Orthopaedics 7(3):51-61, 1983.)

patient. This projection gives the profile view of the posterior column; it in combination with anteroposterior and lateral views enables one to know exactly where the pelvic limbs of the rods lie in the ilia. Sometimes penetration of the ilium can be seen only on this view.

Spinal Arthrodesis

The lumbosacral junction is in an especially opportune location at which to observe the radiographic aspects of spinal arthrodesis. It is possible to get a clear view of the host response to a bone grafting procedure, since the area of intended new bone formation along the lateral gutter and onto the sacrum are not obscured

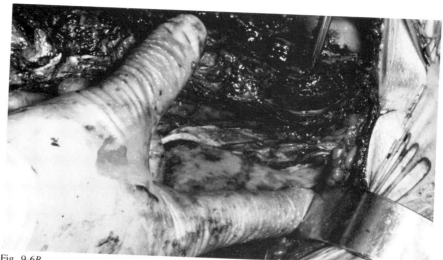

Fig. 9-6*B*.

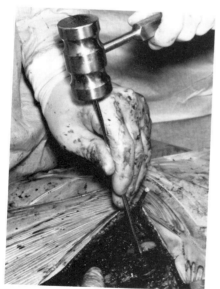

Fig. 9-6*C*.

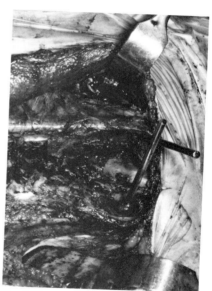

Fig. 9-6*D*.

by superimposed bony structures. On a combination of anteroposterior, lateral, and 45-degree oblique x-ray projections, one can usually see the facet joints and assess their fate. Because the lumbosacral junction has traditionally been a difficult area in which to effect fusion when done in conjunction with scoliosis surgery, it seems probable that techniques that are successful here will be successful in other regions of the spine.

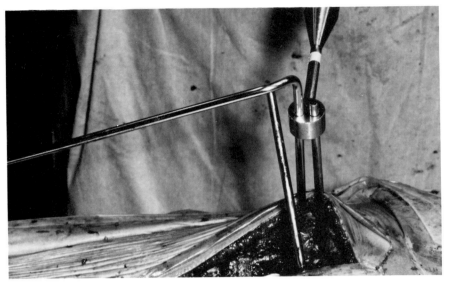

Fig. 9-6*E*.

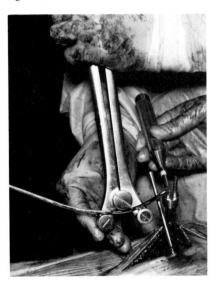

While there is general agreement that the realization of a solid spinal arthrodesis is fundamental to a successful outcome, there is some variation in opinion about what surgical manipulations are essential to achieve this. We know a great deal more about instrumentation of the spine than we do about fusion biology. It seems that most surgeons, us included, have biases concerning fusion techniques and goals which cannot be fully evaluated because of incomplete data bases. The

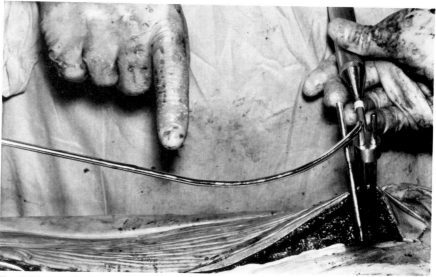

Fig. 9-6*G*.

surgical manipulations done for fusion have come about in a pragmatic, evolutionary way rather than in a scientific manner.

Among the variables one might consider in evaluating a fusion technique are decortication of the spine, excision of the facet joints, type and placement of bone graft, volume of bone graft, quality of immobilization, presence or absence of a metabolic bone disease, pharmacologic effect on new bone formation, and interaction among these variables. From time to time since Russell Hibbs introduced the technique of spinal fusion, the basic concepts and emphasis have drifted one way and then another. In more recent years, the work of Dr. John Moe resulted in a strong belief in the need for decortication and facet excision—a belief adopted and promulgated by Dr. Paul Harrington.[18] One might question the data base underlying Dr. Moe's firm recommendation of these surgical manipulations, however. Decortication was brought forth as a matter of tradition, which was initiated by Hibbs. Dr. Moe's data, based on surgical treatment without instrumentation but with plaster correction and immobilization, showed that in idiopathic scoliosis, facet excision made no difference in the fusion rate; that facet excision yielded a better, but unacceptable-by-today's-standards fusion rate in paralytic deformities; and that the identity of the operating surgeons, inferring the skill of execution of the procedure, was the greatest single factor in successful outcomes.[18] At the time we began to apply the technique of LRI, an arbitrary decision about decortication had to be made. On the one hand, it was traditional, but on the other, it would probably weaken the vertebral lamina appreciably. Since we had been performing posterior cervical spinal arthrodesis for a number of years without decortication, we felt that a review of these cases might give some insight. There were no pseudarthroses in a series of 47 consecutive posterior cervical spine fusions. Is the cervical spine

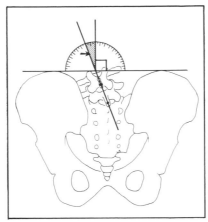

Fig. 9-7A. Angle L4-5P is the angular relationship between a line connecting the spinous processes of L4 and L5 and the perpendicular to a line across the top of the iliac crest. In this example, it is 20 degrees left.

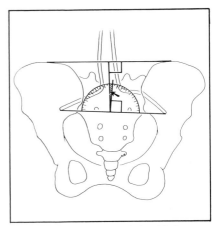

B, Angle IP is the angular relationship between a line perpendicular to a line connecting the tips of the pelvic limbs of the implant and a second perpendicular to a line across the top of the iliac crest. In this example, it is 10 degrees left.

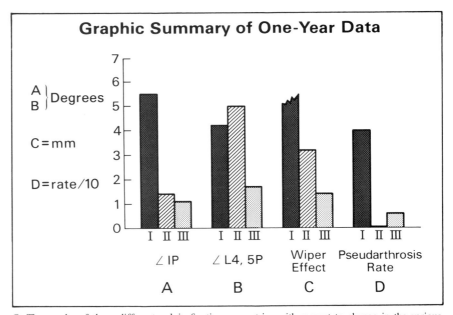

C, The results of three different pelvic fixation geometries with respect to change in the various parameters over a one-year follow-up period is shown. I represents a straight-through Harrington sacral bar type of geometry. II represents a group in which the iliac portions of the implant pass through the posterior column at a depth of six centimeters or greater, but lie greater than 1.5 centimeters cephalad to the sciatic notch. III represents the group in which the iliac portions pass through the posterior column at a depth greater than 6 centimeters and lie within 1.5 centimeters of the sciatic notch.

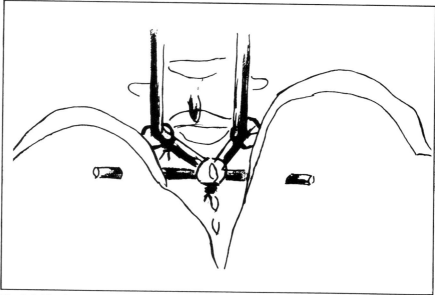

Fig. 9-8. Fixation of the pelvis for cases with good posterior elements and little lateral stress. This technique uses a three-point fixation, crossing the iliac wings with contralateral L-bars and a wire fixation at the S1 facet joints.

biologically different from the thoracic and lumbar spine? We adopted the working hypothesis that it was not; therefore in our technique, no decortication is performed.

What about facet excision? To us, Dr. Moe's data were unconvincing; the cases in which he found it to make a difference were eventually thought to require both an anterior and a posterior arthrodesis with combined Dwyer and Harrington instrumentation, plus postoperative immobilization. We knew that with successful cervical spine fusion, the facets eventually fuse. With successful ischiofemoral fusion, the hip joint undergoes a spontaneous arthrodesis.[1] Why would not the same thing happen in the thoracic and lumbar spine? Our working hypothesis has been that it would. Our present belief is that facet excision probably results in a fusion that gains stiffness more rapidly, but in the face of excellent internal fixation, there is no long-term difference. Effective immobilization probably offsets any gain from facet excision.

Our technique emphasized meticulous cleaning of the spine and addition of a large volume of autogenous bone lateral to the spinal implant. The principles we espouse are: (1) A massive fusion with the largest possible area moment of inertia is a surgical goal; (2) there is a relationship between the volume of the bone graft and the mass of the fusion; (3) fresh, autogenous bone is the best graft material, and (4) excellent fixation is a key requirement for the success of our technique. Following these principles, we accomplished a 96% fusion rate at the lumbosacral junction in scoliosis patients who had no external immobilization.[6] If there is a better technique, hundreds of cases will have to be analyzed to demonstrate it, since the failure rate is so low that any difference would be very small.

Pitfalls

As in any complex surgical undertaking, a number of possible complications may be encountered in performing L-rod instrumentation of a spinal deformity with pelvic fixation. The following list represents the more important ones that experience has bestowed upon us.[5,6]

Inadequate Preoperative Stress Studies

Because the majority of candidates for pelvic fixation have inadequate postural control mechanisms and decompensation, most will need instrumentation from the upper thoracic spine to the pelvis. In these cases, simple bending films are not sufficient for preoperative planning. For example, the relatively rigid thoracolumbar curve may require a compensating thoracic curve to be introduced if T1 is to be centered over the pelvis. Another more problematic example is the patient who has a double curve with the thoracic component being more rigid than the lumbar component. In such a case, correction of each component of the deformity to the greatest extent possible will severely decompensate the patient. What will be required for balance correction is apparent only on stretch films.

We perform our stress studies with the patient either on the Risser table, in a pelvic harness and head halter traction, or on the CircOLectric bed using tong gravity traction and an incline of about 60 degrees. Lateral trunk pressure appropriate to the particular deformity is applied with either method. In this manner, exactly what is needed to effect optimal truncal balance and compensation can be ascertained; the surgical outcome is determined preoperatively.

Asymmetric Pelvis

Although a line across the top of the iliac crest is the traditional guide for judging compensation and balance of the trunk, its use in patients with pelvic asymmetry may be grossly misleading. In our experience, patients who have a paralytic disease, especially poliomyelitis, and those with arthrogryposis involving the pelvic musculature have been the most likely to have an asymmetric pelvis. With such pelvic asymmetry, a true anteroposterior (AP) view of the pelvis will reveal that a line across the bottom of the ischial tuberosities is not parallel to a line drawn across the top of the iliac crest. Since one sits on the ischial tuberosities, balancing the spine with respect to the iliac crest can create an oblique sitting base. We consider it essential to have a true AP x-ray of the pelvis as well as 45-degree oblique outlet views in patients with suspected pelvic asymmetry. If the asymmetry is recognized before surgery, the operation can be planned to provide a square sitting base. The 45-degree oblique outlet views will reveal any bending deformity through the posterior column and transverse bar of the ilium.

Inadequate Exposure

In our experience, the only way we have been able to perform instrumentation of the spine accurately and realize preoperative surgical goals has been to expose both iliac crests widely. It is necessary to have sufficient exposure to identify unequivocally the tops of the iliac crest so that compensation can be measured. We generally use a surgical T-square to do this. Visualization of the sciatic notches is necessary for accurate pin placement.

Sacral Spine Incision

Because it is necessary to work at the lower margin of the posterior superior iliac spines, a long incision that extends over the sacrum is required. At the lower extreme, it is best to curve the skin incision slightly away from the midline so that when the patient is placed supine in the postoperative period, the sacral spines are not pressing directly into the surgical wound. Additionally, in patients with very prominent sacral spines, it helps to trim them to a shorter length.

Accessory Sacroiliac (Ilioaxial) Joints

Normally, there is a narrow gap superior and posterior to the auricular surfaces of the ilium and the sacrum, the interval occupied by the dorsal and interosseous sacral iliac ligaments. In the usual case, the guide pin penetrates the ilium at the level of the lower margin of the posterior superior iliac spine just lateral to the dorsal sacral iliac ligament. In about one-third of patients, accessory sacral iliac or ilioaxial joints are present and may cause some confusion.[5,6,15,22,25] In these instances, synovial joints between the posterior ilium and posterior sacrum are present medial to the interosseous sacral iliac ligaments. If this circumstance is not recognized in a pin tract that is clearly established in the ilium, there is a risk of driving of the pin across the bony gap between the ilium and the sacrum, through the sacroiliac joint, and along the pectineal line inside the pelvis. One clue that this may be happening in surgery is that the pin becomes more vertical as it is being driven. The trochar tip of the pin skates along the medial bony wall of the posterior ilium and into the sacroiliac joint. In cases with accessory sacroiliac joints, one should either drill, curette, or rongeur enough of the iliac entry point to be certain that the pin passes cleanly into the posterior column.

Penetration of the Ilium

In our experience, penetration of the ilium laterally, medially, or inferiorly has led to some loss of pelvic fixation, as manifested by a change in the position of the pelvic segments of the implant relative to the pelvis during the first postoperative year. One of the serious flaws of high placement of pelvic fixation is that the ilium is almost always penetrated when the implant is opposite the membranous portion. Extreme lateral penetration with at least six centimeters of the iliac segment being intraosseous seems to be benign, but more data are needed. Presently, we would accept extreme lateral penetration when recognized at surgery, but would replace the pelvic guide pin if the point of exit is at any other site. Accurate postoperative assessment for pin penetration requires AP, lateral, and 45-degree oblique outlet views of the pelvis. When penetration is not discovered until the postoperative period, it may be wise to place the patient in a plaster cast or brace.

Wiring the First Sacral Lamina

Developing and wiring the first sacral lamina makes no significant contribution to pelvic fixation.[6] It does introduce two significant hazards, however. Because the AP dimension of the sacral neural canal may be small, there is a risk of nerve root contusion and compression. If one feels compelled to wire the sacrum despite this risk, we recommend that a preoperative CAT scan of the sacrum be done. Since epidural fat may be sparse in the sacrum, the risk of lacerating the dura during opening of sacral interlaminar spaces is increased. Furthermore, the sacral dura may be thin and fragile; repair of a dural laceration here can be frustrating. We feel that sacral wiring is best avoided.

Too Long a Sacral Segment

Occasionally, after carefully shaping an L-rod for pelvic fixation, the surgeon will learn upon trial insertion that the sacral segment of the rod is too long, and the bend between the sacral and spinal segments impinges against the base of the sacral spinous processes. The rod can not be inserted properly. One can either adjust the already shaped rod or start afresh. When this happens, we usually make the bend between the spinal and sacral segments less acute and adjust the pelvic end of the implant to fit the angle of sacral inclination as necessary. This adjustment results in a sacral segment that passes more obliquely than usual across the posterior sacral surface, but this seems to make no difference clinically and saves a great deal of operative time.

Inadequate Stiffness of Spinal Segments of Implants

With secure pelvic fixation, it has been possible to recognize that the spinal segments of the implant may bend to some degree in very large individuals or those with severe deformity associated with asymmetric muscle activity in the trunk. Our experience is insufficient to establish a documented solution to this problem. Probably the best approach is to substitute at least one 1/4-inch rod for the usual 3/16-inch rod; in a very large individual, one may consider substituting 1/4-inch rods for each of the 3/16-inch rods. Presently, biomechanical studies are underway to define further and hopefully develop an appropriate means of solving this problem.[26]

Extension Contractures of the Hip

It is crucial that extension contractures of the hips be recognized and dealt with before connecting the spine to the pelvis with LRI. Otherwise, when the patient with such contractures attempts to sit, the spinal implant may fracture the pelvis. When the contractures are not recognized until after the spinal surgery, either the patient should not sit until arthrodesis is assured or the contractures should be surgically relieved.

Closure

The scoliosis patient who needs spinal arthrodesis extending to the sacrum challenges one's surgical techniques and judgment. By eliminating the need for postoperative immobilization, L-rod instrumentation has greatly reduced the morbidity of this surgical undertaking. Consequently, the procedure is being much more widely used to solve neuromuscular and lumbosacral scoliosis. Accurate assessment of the problem, thorough preoperative planning, and keen execution of technique are the keys to successful outcome.

Editor's Commentary

There is no doubt that in all existing spinal instrumentation techniques, the weak link has always been the pelvic fixation. Biomechanically, it is quite obvious that when one arthrodeses the lumbar spine, he is not only establishing a long lever arm but is also dealing with lateral (AP), axial (postural curves), and rotational deformities. There is also a very wide biomechanical configuration of S1-L5 that is ideal for movement, although limited in all directions. On the other hand, at the caudal end, the sacrum is triangular and composed of soft bone except at the facet site. Although an excellent cornerstone for closing the pelvic ring, it is tremendously inadequate as a base for a corrective upright column. The immediate joints on either side (the sacroiliacs), although semi-atrophic and half joints, are broad and well supplied by sacral nerve endings. The ilium, mostly spongy bone, offers a poor place for "bone metal" fixation.

The question that remains unanswered is what will be the role of methyl methacrylate or another "filler" under these conditions of poor bony substance fixation. The Galveston pelvic fixation remains an important contribution to SSI, especially in individuals that have large posterior element defects. There are several problems with the technique, however. First, it is technically difficult, and it must be individualized. There is no way that a formula can be drawn up for all ages and all disorders. Second, it crosses the sacroiliac joint, making it a stabilizer over a nonarthrodesed joint. Third, it does not cross over to form a coupled force with the contralateral bar. Fourth, the area of fixation in the pelvis in many cases consists of a very thin cortex and deficient spongy bone. Finally, a set length cannot be used.

Its advantages are obvious and adequately pointed out in this chapter. The ideal would be fixation through two good cortices with three points of fixation on either side, broad enough to control the entire pelvis. We have found that for the routine case with good posterior elements and mainly postural strains, crossed bars over the S1-S2 interspace through the two cortices of the contralateral iliac wings, and wired in at both the S1 facet joints and the junction of S1 and S2, give adequate fixation and are technically easy to execute (Fig. 9-8).

Surgical experience with SSI must be evaluated continuously, because what is good for one condition is not necessarily good for something else. In my own surgical experience with fixation to the pelvis in neuromuscular cases (including paraplegics), we have reviewed a total of 93 cases after a two- to four-year follow-up. Forty-one were growing children without arthrodesis and transiliac fixation. Of these, only two cases were cut out of the ilium; eight other cases showed movement with the pelvic fixation; and sixteen had a normal loss of correction one year postoperatively due to growth. All still had movement at L5-S1 in flexion, but there were no instrument failures.

In the second group of 52 patients treated with an arthrodesis through S1, no immobilization was used postoperatively. The fixation was again transilium (Fig. 9-8). Arthrodesis included facetectomies, decortication, and posterolateral bone grafting over the transverse processes. There were no cases with more than 30° of pelvic obliquity in this group, who underwent only a posterior procedure. The overall correction was 73%, obtained by direct lateral bend and fixed by SSI. There was one broken rod in this group, no wire fatigue, and no recognizable pseudarthrosis. All these patients were treated without external fixation, but all had limited physical activity during their first six months postoperatively.

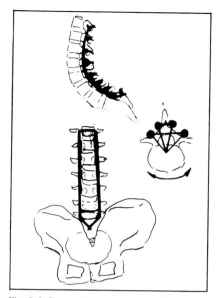

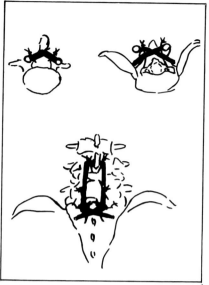

Fig. 9-9. For rotational deformities, it is important to put the bars as far laterally or forward as possible, so as to make an equilateral triangle with the middle column in the axial plane. One may also conserve the normal lordosis and not cross the sacroiliac joints, which will become painful in adults.

Fig. 9-10. With adequate segmental wiring, rectangular rods bent to fit the cephalad lamina and dovetailed caudally to fit the sacrum provide a good fixation in distraction for a limited number of segments.

For rotational deformities like lumbar fractures and degenerative spondylolisthesis, use of an inverted dovetail that fits snugly against the S1 facet and is securely fastened to the S1-S2 lamina avoids recurrence of the deformity. It is a weak fixation for either flexion or extension forces or for pelvic obliquity, however (Fig. 9-9).

Forty-three cases of rotational deformities have been studied, with an average follow-up of 16 months. Thirty cases that underwent routine SSI including Galveston fixation experienced recurrence to different degrees, even if the patients remained asymptomatic. The remaining 13 cases, which have the shortest follow-up (average of 13 months), have shown no recurrence of the deformity and no pseudarthrosis. These patients received an SSI fixation as illustrated in Fig. 9-9. All seven fracture cases were treated with external immobilization postoperatively. For short lumbar arthrodesis, including the occasional child, a rectangular rod with dovetailed sacral ends produces excellent flexion-extension immobilization and can maintain distraction over a short area of the spine (Fig. 9-10).

Square rods with or without sacral dovetails have been used by us since 1976 for fixation of the low back. Of 132 cases reviewed with arthrodesis from S1 to L5 or L4, with an average follow-up of 50 months, only five cases were found to have

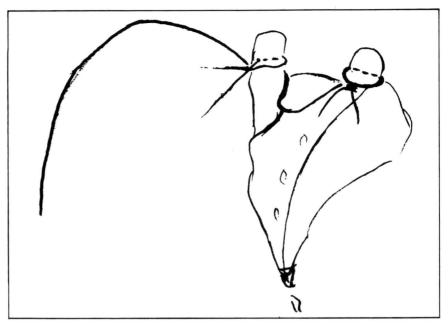

Fig. 9-11. There are two good ways of holding on the S1 facet. On the left, this is accomplished by drilling a hole through the outer edge and looping the remaining articular process. On the right, a complete loop of the S1 articular process is done.

pseudarthrosis. Two additional cases had instrumentation failure (broken rods) with no symptoms and no provable osseous mass defect on x-ray films. Only ten patients in this group used a brace postoperatively for a period of three months.

Both of these last two methods have the great advantage of not crossing the lumbosacral joint, which in our experience has been a source of prolonged rehabilitation in the adult patient.

In all pelvic fixations, I have found that except for infralaminar wire loops in S1, S2, or both, the best bone substance is at the facet of S1-L5 and should be used as one point of fixation bilaterally. Holding on to the S1 facet can be done either by looping the entire facet or by transfixing it, providing three-point fixation bilaterally (Fig. 9-11). All in all, as in other aspects of SSI, this part of the technique cannot be put into dogmatic terms and must be individualized and tailored to each patient.

References

1. Adams JC: Ischio-Femoral Arthrodesis. Baltimore, MD, Williams and Wilkins Co., 1966, p 37.

2. Allen BL Jr, Ferguson RL: L-rod instrumentation for scoliosis in cerebral palsy. J Pediatr Ortho 2:87-96, 1982.

3. Allen BL Jr, Ferguson RL: The operative treatment of myelomeningocele spine deformity—1979. Ortho Clin North Am 10:845-861, 1979.

4. Allen BL Jr, Ferguson RL: The Galveston technique for L-rod instrumentation of the scoliotic spine. Spine 7:276-284, 1982.

5. Allen BL Jr, Ferguson RL: A pictorial guide to the Galveston LRI pelvic fixation technique. Cont Ortho 7:51-61, 1983.

6. Allen BL Jr, Ferguson RL: The Galveston technique of pelvic fixation with L-rod instrumentation of the spine. Spine (*in press*)

7. Black J, Martin EC, Gelman H, and Morris DM: Serum concentrations of chromium, cobalt and nickel after total hip replacement. Biomaterials (*in press*).

8. Bonnett C, Brown JC, Grow T: Thoracolumbar scoliosis in cerebral palsy. J Bone Jt Surg 58A:328-336, 1976.

9. Broadstone P, Leatherman KD: Consider postoperative immobilization of double L-rod segmental spinal instrumentation. Proceedings of the Scoliosis Research Society, New Orleans, 1983.

10. Brown JC, Swank WM, Specht L: Combined anterior and posterior spine fusion in cerebral palsy. Spine 7:570-573, 1982.

11. Ferguson RL, Allen BL Jr: The technique of scoliosis revision surgery utilizing L-rod instrumentation. J Pediatr Ortho (*in press*).

12. Ferguson RL, Allen BL Jr: Staged correction of neuromuscular scoliosis. J Pediatr Ortho (*in press*).

13. Fisk JR, Winter RB, Moe JH: The lumbosacral curve in idiopathic scoliosis. J Bone Jt Surg 62A:39-46, 1980.

14. Floman Y, Michaeli LJ, Penny JN, Riseborough EJ, Hall JE: Combined anterior and posterior fusion in seventy-three spinally deformed patients. Clin Ortho 164:110-122, 1982.

15. Hadley LA: Accessory sacroiliac articulations. J Bone Jt Surg 34A:149-155, 1952.

16. Harrington PR: Technical details in relation to the successful use of instrumentation in scoliosis. Ortho Clin North Am 3:49-67, 1972.

17. Memoli VA, Woodman JL, Urban RM, Galante JO: Malignant neoplasms associated with orthopaedic implant materials. Proceedings of the Orthopaedic Research Society, New Orleans, 1982.

18. Moe JH: A critical analysis of fusion for scoliosis. J Bone Jt Surg 40A:529-554, 1958.

19. O'Brien JP, Yau ACMC: Anterior and posterior correction and fusion for paralytic scoliosis. Clin Ortho 86:151-153, 1972.

20. O'Brien JP, Dwyer AP, Hodgson AR: Paralytic pelvic obliquity. J Bone Jt Surg 57A:626-631, 1975.

21. O'Brien JP, Yau ACMC, Fertzbein S, Hodgson AR: Combined staged anterior and posterior correction and fusion of the spine in scoliosis following poliomyelitis. Clin Ortho 110:81-89, 1975.

22. Peterson OVCE: Uber Articulations Flachen an der Hinterflache des Os Sacrum. Anat Anzeig 26:521-524, 1905.

23. Stanitski CL, Micheli LJ, Hall JE, Rosenthal RK: Surgical correction of spinal deformity in cerebral palsy. Spine 7:563-569, 1982.

24. Swank SM, Brown JC, Williams L, Stark E: Spinal fusion using Zielke instrumentation—a preliminary report. Ortho 5:1172-1182, 1982.

25. Trotter M: A common anatomical variation in the sacroiliac region. J Bone Jt Surg 22:293-299, 1940.

26. Weiler PJ: Buckling analysis of spinal implant devices used for the surgical treatment of scoliosis. Thesis, University of Waterloo, Waterloo, Ontario, Canada, 1983.

27. Woodman JL, Memoli VA, Urban RM, Galante JO: Nickel and titanium release in a carcinogenesis study of orthopaedic implant materials. Proceedings of the Orthopaedic Research Society, Anaheim, CA, 1983.

Eggshell Procedure

10

SPINAL SURGERY HAS MADE TREMENDOUS advances in the past few years. Initially, the surgeon attacked spinal deformities strictly from the posterior approach. Often, severe rigid deformities could be altered very little, and if extreme force was used, the incidence of complications was high. For example, the kyphotic rheumatoid spine was treated with a closed wedged osteotomy, posterior to the roots. With sufficient force, this wedge was closed by rupturing both the discs anteriorly and the anterior longitudinal ligament, or by interbody fracture. In the older patient, this frequently put a great deal of tension on the anterior structures. Eventually, anterior procedures for severe rigid spinal deformities were used. Again, many of these allowed only partial correction because the posterior and anterior structures were not being attacked at the same time. Thus, fixation placed anteriorly gave less than desirable correction and occasionally resulted in three-stage procedures. The patient had posterior loosening, anterior loosening, and, finally, posterior stabilization.

In the beginning, one-stage procedures were plagued by complications and ceased to be popular. With our newer technology, it appeared that a one-stage correction of certain rigid deformities could be done if the cord and vascular structures could be protected. Thus, about ten years ago, the author started doing decancellization procedures, carried out from posteriorly. The principle was to weaken the vertebra anterior to the cord, remove all or part of the posterior elements, and produce a controlled compression fracture, while observing the cord and roots. The closing wedge osteotomy used the anterior longitudinal ligament as a hinge. It was essential to be certain that the cord would not be compressed posteriorly by the edges of the posterior elements as they were approximated. There should be no bone left immediately anterior to the neural canal that could buckle into the cord or roots.

It would appear that if such a technique could be evolved for the safe correction of scoliosis, kyphosis, or lordosis, or any combination of these curves, this would be most desirable.

Logic would dictate that the surgeon should keep his eye on the cord, and thus do a laminectomy as the first step. The surgeon would know where he was. Unfortunately, here logic and the cold world separate, for once the roof is lifted on the dura, the cord is exposed to drying and temperature changes and is fair game for misdirected suction, cautery, or instrument.

Indications

The eggshell procedure is designed for the spinal surgeon who plays with spinal bones daily, who has studied the deformity with regular x-rays, myelograms, tomograms, CT scans, and now, perhaps, NMR. When he knows exactly what the bones will look like, then he should operate on them. An ideal case for the procedure would be a congenital short but acute kyphotic deformity of T12 that one would like to correct 40 or 50 degrees. Another deformity might be the acquired postoperative fractured spine that underwent the older procedure of decompressive laminectomy for three levels, with or without stabilization, and has tended to collapse further over the ensuing five to twenty years. The resulting increase in kyphosis may lead to anterior cord compression.

Another deformity is congenital hemivertebra which may be removed, collapsed, or, in the very young, enucleated and the epiphysis fused to allow for slow correction with growth. The procedure is also a satisfactory adjunct for treatment of a spinal fracture in which the surgeon wishes to remove the bone from the canal anterior to the cord without going through the chest. The surgeon is able to stabilize the fracture posteriorly and at the same time decompress the cord anteriorly. Many surgeons do not feel comfortable with an anterior approach.

This technique, like almost every operation in medicine, must give due credit to others. Dr. Arthur Michele and Dr. Frederick J. Krudger described a similar approach in 1949 in "A Surgical Approach to the Vertebral Body."[1] They used the procedure primarily for biopsy of vertebral body lesions. They pointed out the anatomic pathway of going down the pedicle into the body. This permitted abscesses to be drained away from the dura. Bloody lesions could be capped like an

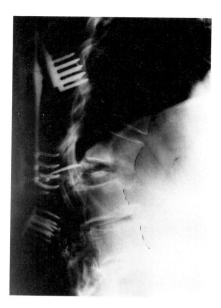

Fig. 10-1. Lateral view of a spine with a marker in place accurately establishing the level of the osteotomy.

oilwell by simply putting a plug of bone or bonewax in the opening of the pedicle to control the bleeding. It thus seemed logical to adapt the vertebral excision from this approach.

Surgical Technique

It is necessary to have an adequate exposure of the deformity. The interval between the lateral margin of the facet and the transverse process must be identified accurately on one or both sides, depending on the nature of the deformity to be corrected. This technique has not been used above C7 because of the vertebral artery and the smallness of the structures. It has been used in all other segments of the spine, including the upper segment of the sacrum.

The desired vertebra is selected and accurately identified on x-ray examination (Fig. 10-1). The interval between the pedicle and transverse process is decorticated using a small curette. Cancellous bone is then carefully removed from the pedicle (Fig. 10-2). This is easier to do at the level at L5, where the pedicles are very large, than it is D5, where one must be very careful.

When previous surgery has been carried out, especially with old fractures, it may be necessary to drill through the sclerotic bone with a hand drill. The bit should be hand tightened in the chuck, so that the surgeon knows when it catches

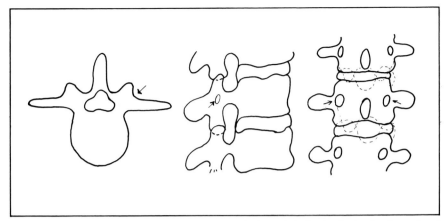

Fig. 10-2. Anteroposterior, lateral, and cross-sectional views of the lumbar body, showing point of entrance over the pedicle.

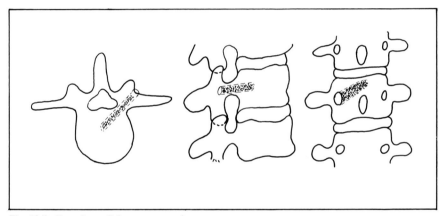

Fig. 10-3. How the pedicles are curetted.

hold of one of the cortices. It is very important to stay inside the cortices, especially superiorly, medially, and inferiorly. One does not want to wander laterally very much either, or one will be plagued by troublesome and needless bleeding from the segmental vertebral vessels. There is surprisingly little bleeding from the inside of the vertebra. Should one encounter a large sinus, one simply presses bone wax into the sinuses and directs one's curette elsewhere.

The course of the curette is directed downward and medially under the cord at a 45-degree angle until one has gone halfway under the cord (Fig. 10-3). Then one goes to the opposite side of the table and repeats the process from that side, until the two tunnels meet (Fig. 10-4). At this point, it is advisable for the first few operations to confirm one's location. The surgeon will usually find himself halfway

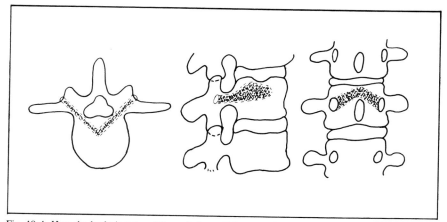

Fig. 10-4. How the body is entered through the pedicles, care being taken to preserve the walls, thus protecting the cord and nerve roots. The excavation of both pedicles going down into the body is shown.

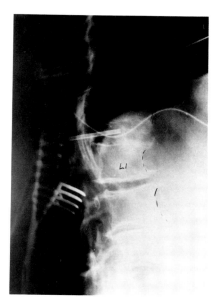

Fig. 10-5. An x-ray probe halfway into the vertebral body.

through the vertebra and about one centimeter anterior to the cord (Fig. 10-5).

The procedure now becomes simple for a while. One doctor excavates cancellous bone with long No. 1, No. 3, or No. 5 curettes, while the assistant removes the loose bone from the other side with a small pituitary or forceps (Fig. 10-6). The light must be directed into the tunnels from each side. The assistant keeps the base of the tunnels dry with suction. Usually, at this point, the curette is directed upward to remove the vertebral and end-plate, and the disk is identified and curetted out (Fig. 10-7). One may then crack the transverse process downward and

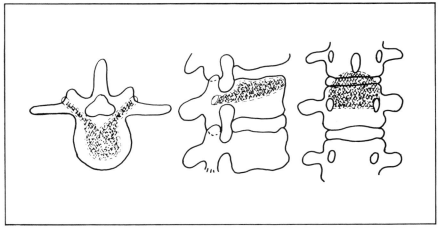

Fig. 10-6. More material has been removed, leaving the body more as an eggshell.

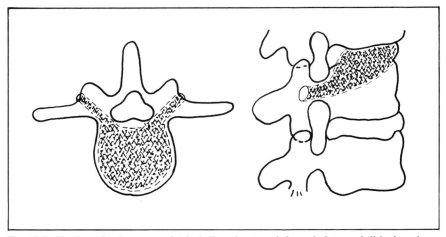

Fig. 10-7. The bone is almost completely hollowed out, and the end-plates and disks have been removed.

remove the base of a rib in the dorsal spine partially or totally, to permit the "roof of the cave" one has created to be thinned down. Under direct vision, the bone is removed from under the anterior longitudinal ligament until it is the thickness of an eggshell (Fig. 10-8).

At this time, it is desirable to dissect carefully subperiosteally along the enucleated body, directly anterior to the transverse process. With a thin-billed rongeur, a strip of bone is removed from either side of the vertebral body so that when one is ready to crush the body, the line has already been started at least halfway around the vertebra. This is very much like scoring a piece of glass prior to breaking it. With careful dissection, one does not need to create bleeding while doing this.

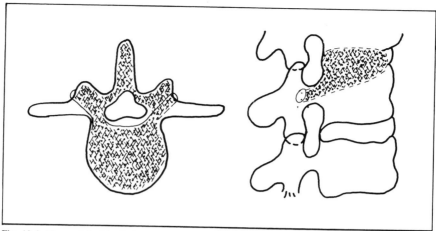

Fig. 10-8. The vertebral body is ready to be collapsed.

During this portion of the operation, the cord and roots have been protected from drying and the trauma associated with bone removal. Bleeding has been minimal. Next, the surgeon must decide what type of instrumentation, if any, he wishes to use and prepare for its insertion.

For example, if one were going to do an epiphyseodesis on a very small child, one would simply bone graft the end-plates and use no metallic implant. If one were to replace a tumor body, one might fill the cavity with bone cement. If the problem was an older child with a hemivertebra, one might use a small Knodt rod, compress the deformity, and place a small amount of bone graft anteriorly. If this were a kyphotic or scoliotic deformity, closed loop or U-shaped contoured segmental fixation could be used very nicely (Figs. 10-9 and 10-10). Compression rodding of the Harrington variety may be used by the surgeon who, after doing all this, fears the placing of sublaminar wires for SSI.

Again, we emphasize that before one exposes the cord, he should prepare the areas above and below the osteotomy in order to reduce the time that the cord and roots are exposed to the elements and to the possible trauma of instrumentation and suction.

Once everything is set for the placement of the fixation, one should remove the spinous process and lamina either totally or partially, depending on the deformity and the degree of correction one desires. Next, the lateral walls of the pedicles are caved outward with a long sharp curette or "joker," or are rongeured away. The cord must be protected from trauma at all times. The last step is to take a long "joker," place it under the cord carefully, and cave the roof of the eggshelled vertebra into the excavated body (Fig. 10-11). At this time, one places any soft cancellous bone back in the cavity if one feels the need, closes the wedge slowly, and secures the fixation. Fig. 10-12 illustrates the vertebral bodies being excavated. At this time, the narcotic anesthetic is reversed. It usually takes approximately two to five minutes for the wake-up test to be performed. The remainder of the spine is

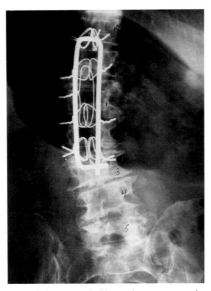
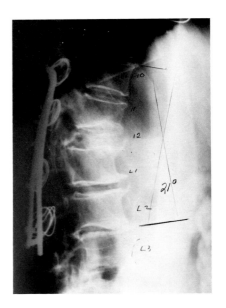

Figs. 10-9 and 10-10. X-rays in anteroposterior and lateral views with the instrumentation in place—in this case, a closed loop Luque rod.

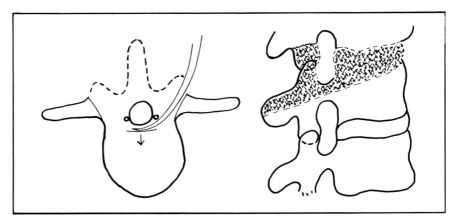

Fig. 10-11. The "joker" in place ready to collapse the eggshell, after the posterior elements have been removed and the pedicles have been collapsed outward.

bone grafted from the iliac crest, and the wound is closed. Appropriate postoperative care is then instituted.

So far, this procedure has been carried out successfully in more than 25 cases in the past ten years in neurologically intact individuals without causing paralysis. It has been used in the neurologically incomplete individual without increasing paralysis. A variation of this procedure has been used for numerous acute fractures

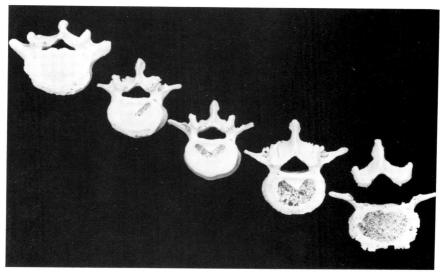

Fig. 10-12. Five vertebral bodies in the actual stages of dissection.

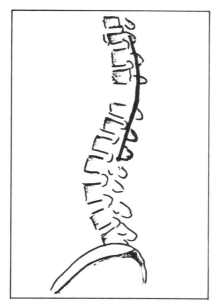

Fig. 10-13. A total vertebrectomy means extirpation of the vertebral body and all the posterior osseous vertebral elements. In this figure, it is maintained by a molded posterior double rod.

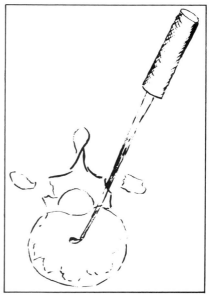

Fig. 10-14. The eggshell procedure as modified by Dr. Heinig is shown, taking all the cancellous bone from the vertebral body through the pedicle with a curette in preparation for corrective collapse.

in which bone fragments are removed or repositioned at the time of stabilization. This is accomplished by simply going down the pedicle and getting to the floor of the vertebra by this approach.

This is a safe procedure in the hands of the proficient spine surgeon who can avoid the temptation of locating the cord first. The success of the procedure is inversely proportional to the time the cord is exposed to the sight of the surgeon and his associates.

Editor's Commentary

Dr. Heinig's modification of the Michele and Frederick approach to the anterior vertebral body has improved our possibilities of correcting spinal pathology. One of the most important principals developed as a result of the use of SSI is correction of the deformity by shortening procedures without causing undue force from the instrumentation. This has been well established in the eggshell procedure.

In general orthopedics, shortening of a deformed bone is the most common way to correct a deformity and the most common way to induce an arthrodesis. In severe deformities of the spine for which any corrective procedure produces lengthening, maximum relaxation of the intervertebral arteries and the anterior longitudinal artery is a safety measure worth taking. If the osseous deformity is not destroyed, it will limit the correction, as will the relative flexibility of the intervertebral spaces and the vascular supply to the neural cord and to soft tissue contractures.

The limitation of shortening procedures is that they produce disruption of the neurologic components, disruption of the blood supply to the neural cord, and soft tissue contractures on the contralateral side. Shortening procedures include: (1) closed-wedge osteotomies of the posterior elements, (2) diskectomies, (3) corpectomies, and (4) vertebrectomies.

Indications for Shortening Procedures

The indications for *posterior osteotomies* are: (1) correction of scoliosis, (2) correction of kyphosis (posterior closing wedge), and (3) correction of lordosis (destruction of posterior deformity).

The indications for *diskectomy* are to produce: (1) segmental flexibility, (2) correction of anterior deformity, and (3) anterior fusion under compression (kyphosis).

The primary indication for *corpectomy* is to destroy anterior deformity or to

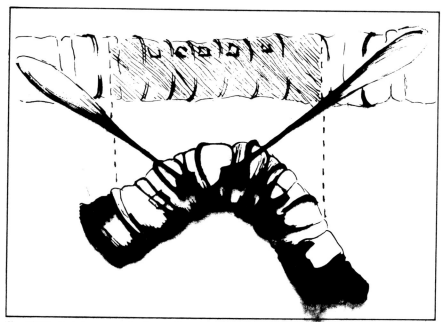

Fig. 10-15. Anterior removal of cancellous bone and disks without interfering with intervertebral segmental vessels. Note small disk sites.

do anterior decompression of the neural canal. Multiple corpectomies for removal of tumors or infection are in fact shortening procedures, but care must be taken not to collapse the spinal column and interfere with the blood supply to the nerve cord. This is always a danger.

The indications for *vertebrectomy* are essentially severe deformities, either in the AP plane, in the axial plane, or in the segmental plane.

Vertebrectomy Technique

Vertebrectomy can be done by total extirpation, as for an infection, a tumor or congenital defects (Fig. 10-13). Posterior decancellation for correction of burst fractures or acute kyphosis and spondylolisthesis (eggshell procedure) can also be done (Fig. 10-14). Finally, an anterior diskectomy and decancellation procedure can be used to produce a sausage-like tubular structure, which is actually periosteum with all the segmental vessels intact and stuffed with cancellous bone. This is an ideal osteogenic situation (Fig. 10-15).

In cases of extreme deformity, it might be necessary to do multiple vertebrectomies to realign or transpose the spine toward the midline. The obvious danger is the elimination of the blood supply to the neural cord from tying the segmental vessels in the anterior approach and two weeks later causing a second insult to the

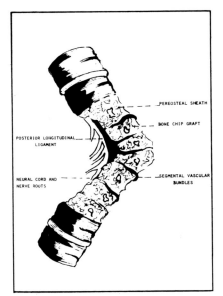

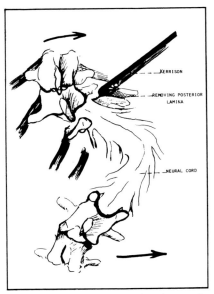

Fig. 10-16. After total decancellation procedures of multiple vertebrae have been done from an anterior approach, bony chips are replaced into the periosteal sheath. The segmental vascular bundle and the posterior neural elements are respected.

Fig. 10-17. Removal of posterior elements in second stage procedure should only be done to: (1) obtain maximum alignment, (2) relax the neural cord, or (3) avoid nerve entrapment.

vascular supply of the nerve cord by doing multiple laminectomies and pedilectomies. For this reason, we have adapted the eggshell procedure to an anterior approach—transthoracic or retroperitoneal.[2]

Total multiple vertebrectomy is usually done in two stages. In the first stage, the diskectomies, decancellation, and mobilizing procedures are done though small apertures at the disk site, in this way leaving the segmental blood vessels intact. Once all the cancellous bone has been extirpated from the vertebral body, the physician induces greenstick fractures of the cortex. The cancellous bone is replaced, and the disk apertures are closed over with periosteum (Fig. 10-16).

In the second stage, after subperiosteal dissection of the entire deformity, facetectomy is done with partial laminectomy. Flexibility of the deformity is checked. If alignment is not satisfactory, eggshell-type excavation can be done through the pedicles at several levels. This unites the anterior decancellation procedure with the posterior pedicular excavation. Only after being convinced that total removal of the lamina, transverse process, spinous process, and pedicles will give better correction relaxation of the cord or will avoid nerve root involvement should the posterior elements be removed (Fig. 10-17). At this point, extreme care

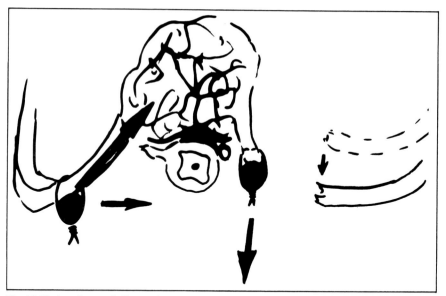

Fig. 10-18. Anterior eggshell procedure has been done (extirpation of the posterior vertebral elements). Osteotomy of the concave rib and osteotomy of the convex transverse process permit derotation of the thoracic ring.

must be taken, because the nerve cord and its corresponding nerve roots will be totally exposed over the area of the vertebrectomy. Continuous irrigation with isotonic solution at body temperature should be used at all times.

The maximum goal of a multiple vertebrectomy is to produce total correction of deformity on either the AP, axial, or segmental level. Sometimes this is not convenient, so a physiologic balance should be accepted. The major restriction in multiple vertebrectomy correction is the structures circumscribing the spinal column, ribs, muscles, and anterior secondary deformities of the sternum and other anterior bony or muscle structures.

To correct thoracic rib hump deformities, it is necessary to osteotomize the concave ribs at the apex, and to osteotomize the transverse process on the convex ribs at the same levels. This will permit: (1) transposition of the neural canal toward the midline of the body, (2) a derotation of the apex of the deformity, and (3) a derotation of the thoracic deformity, lowering the convex rib hump and elevating the concave side (Fig. 10-18). SSI should be done at this second stage. More than as a corrective procedure, however, it should be used as an alignment device and as a fixation instrumentation. It is important to note that a C-bar or rectangular bar must be used to maintain length, and absolutely no distraction should be used. Total three-dimensional segmental balance must be obtained. Decortication and para-vertebral bone graft are laid in contact to produce a 180° fusion mass.

References

1. Michele A, Krudger FJ: A surgical approach to the vertebral body. J Bone Jt Surg 31A:873-878, 1949.
2. Luque ER: Vertebral column transposition. Orthopaedic transaction. J Bone Jt Surg 7(1):29, Spring, 1983.

Application of SSI
to the Lumbosacral Spine

11

Introduction

There are a variety of problems in the lumbar spine that would benefit from a satisfactory method of internal stabilization. Multiple-level fusions have a high incidence of pseudarthrosis, and until now methods such as Harrington instrumentation have been inherently unstable, since they provide attachment only at the ends of the rod systems, in an area where mechanical forces are extreme.

Luque has adapted his unique form of segmental instrumentation to this area of the spine. There is now reason to be optimistic about the use of this system in the management of "problem backs."

The design of the Luque instrumentation for the lumbar spine is still undergoing changes. The current design is either a rectangular or a "dove-tail" configuration, attaching to the sacrum, and has the theoretical advantage of resisting rotational strains.

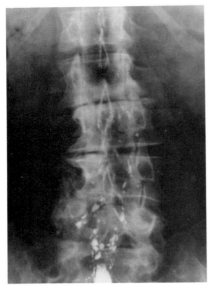 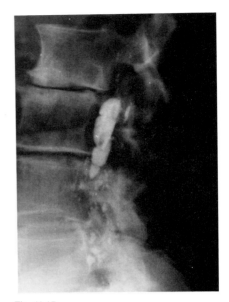

Figs. 11-1A & B. Multiple-level disk degeneration.   Fig. 11-1B.

Indications

Multiple-Level Disc Degeneration (Fig. 11-1)

A single-level fusion has a high incidence of success and does not as a rule require additional stabilization. However, the increased rate of pseudarthrosis with multiple-level fusions warrants consideration of segmental stabilization. Long-term results of SSI are not yet available.

Stabilization After Decompressive Laminectomies for Spinal Stenosis

The aging spine shows progressive overgrowth of the facet joints, particularly involving the superior facet. This produces symptoms of spinal stenosis, which may be either central or lateral (Fig. 11-2). After thorough decompressive laminectomy, the patient's symptoms of claudication are usually relieved, but many patients are required to wear a back brace to prevent pain on movement of the spine. If it is felt that there is significant instability following the wide laminectomy, the

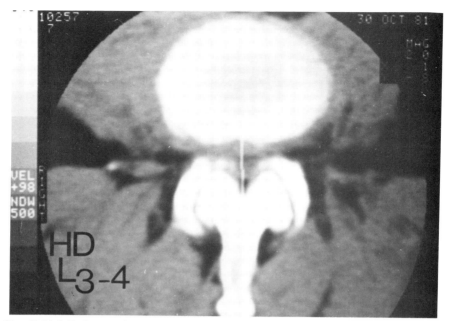

Figs. 11-2*A* & *B*. Severe spinal stenosis.

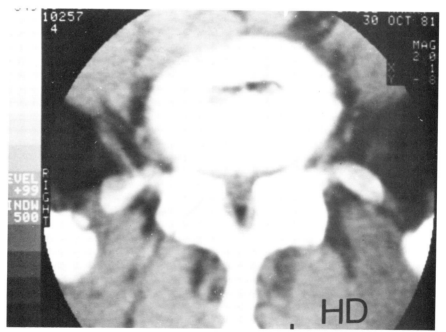

Fig. 11-2*B*.

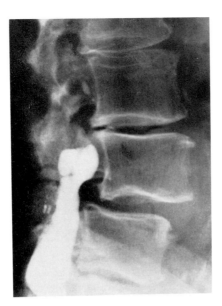

Fig. 11-3*A*. Degenerative spondylolisthesis.

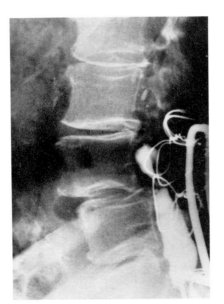
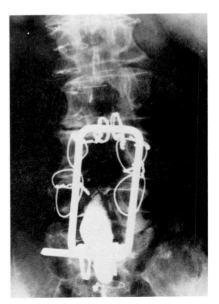

Figs. 11-3*B* & *C*. SSI following laminectomy. (Note: this form of pedicle wire attachment is no longer used.)

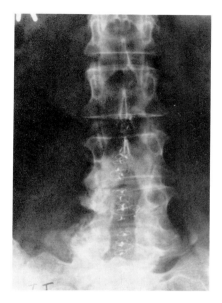

Figs. 11-4*A* & *B*. Previous laminectomy with instability.

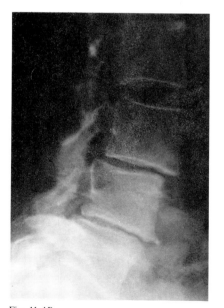

Fig. 11-4*B*.

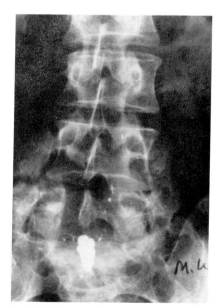

Fig. 11-4*C*. Pseudarthrosis.

SSI system is indicated at the time of the decompressive surgery. Subsequent surgery is technically more difficult owing to the formation of scar tissue.

Degenerative Spondylolisthesis (Fig. 11-3A)

This occurs frequently at the L4-L5 level, where the L5 root is compressed by the inferior lamina of L4, particularly in flexion. If the subluxation does not reduce easily in the extended position, a laminectomy may be required, because the addition of sublaminar wires could cause further compromise of the canal. The rod system is fixated to the lamina at the level above the laminectomy, and to the facet joint at the level of the laminectomy itself (Fig. 11-3B and C). This should prevent further slipping.

Failed Spinal Surgery

The back that has been operated on several times may benefit from segmental stabilization, particularly if there is a pseudarthrosis from a previously attempted fusion (Fig. 11-4). Instability may also be present owing to a previous wide disc removal or damage to the pars interarticularis.

Tumor

Either primary or metastatic tumors involving the lumbar spine can be stabilized to the sacrum using the same rod configuration. This allows the patient freedom of activity as well as significant relief of pain.

Technical Aspects of SSI Application

Positioning of the Patient

The patient is usually placed on an ordinary laminectomy frame with the hip extended to avoid loss of lumbar lordosis. It should be possible to alter the position of the patient into further extension or flexion during surgery.

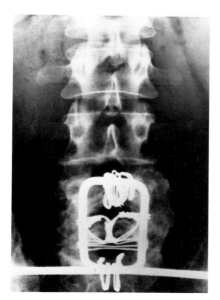

Fig. 11-5A. Original Q-shaped configuration. (No longer used.)

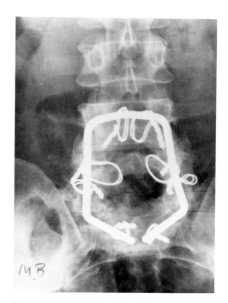

Fig. 11-5B. Dovetail configuration.

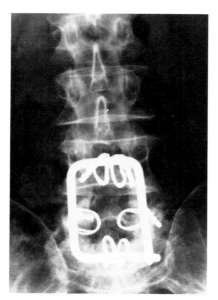

Fig. 11-5C. Rectangular configuration.

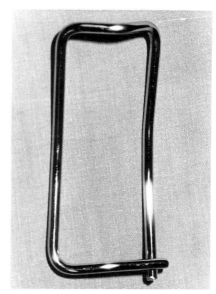

Fig. 11-5D. Contoured rectangular implant.

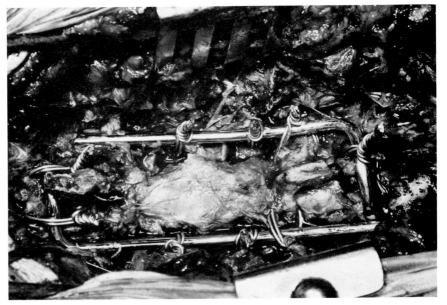

Fig. 11-6. Rectangular implant for multiple-level laminectomy.

Configuration of the Rod

The original design by Luque was that of a Q-shaped rod with horizontal portions penetrating the iliac crests on either side, just above the sacroiliac joint (Fig. 11-5A). This was found to produce radiating pain into the posterior thigh, presumably due to the fact that the rods crossed the sacroiliac joint. This has been altered to the present dove-tail or rectangular shape, which fits closely to the back of the sacrum (Fig. 11-5B to D).

Accurate measurements of the length and width of the rod are made intraoperatively, and the rod is then shaped so that the transverse portion comes to lie directly over the lamina at the upper end. The rod is contoured to it and over the dorsum of the sacrum at its lower end, where it is also contoured (Fig. 11-6). The vertical portions overlie the facet joints. Commonly, ³⁄₁₆-inch rod is used, but obese patients may require the use of the quarter-inch rod.

Attachment to the Spine and Pelvis

For laminar fixation, double wires are passed under the lamina from below upward in the midportion, after excision of the ligamentum flavum on either side of the

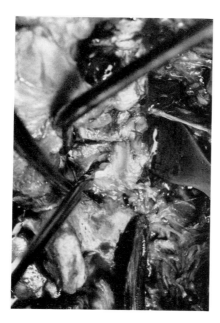

Fig. 11-7. Facet drilling (45-degree angle) for wire placement.

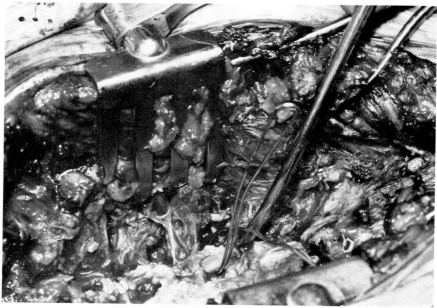

Fig. 11-8. Wire in place.

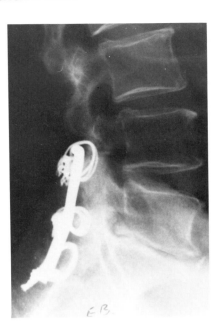

Fig. 11-9. Implant contoured into lordosis.

lamina. The wires are then positioned away from the midline to be tied over the rod to prevent rotation. Sharp ends of wire should never be passed under the lamina. When a double wire is tightened, one must be certain that both portions are equally tight, so that a loop of wire is not left encroaching on the spinal canal.

The lower portion of the rod is anchored to the sacrum through the superior sacral facet, which is usually a strong structure. If the L5 lamina has been previously removed, a drill hole is made through the central portion of the articular surface at about a 45° angle downward and laterally (Fig. 11-7). The L5 root is protected during this maneuver, and double wires are then passed through this hole, to be tied around the rod system (Fig. 11-8).

If the lamina is intact, and there is sufficient room under the lamina, either a double or single wire may be used to provide laminar attachment. At other levels, if a laminectomy has been carried out, a similar hole is made with the drill pointing downward and laterally from the medial side of the facet, to exit just above the base of the transverse process. Previous attempts at wire fixation around the superior facet in the form of a loop passed under the medial portion of the facet in the form of a loop passed under the medial portion of the facet were associated with incidences of increased neurologic deficit of a transient nature. This has been abandoned. (See Fig. 11-3B and C.)

The sacral canal should be assessed preoperatively to determine whether the depth is adequate to allow passage of a wire under the S1 lamina. This can be evaluated by a CT scan and myelography and also by visualization at the time of surgery, when actual measurement of the depth can be carried out. A central drill hole may be made between the lamina of S1 and S2 for the passage of wires.

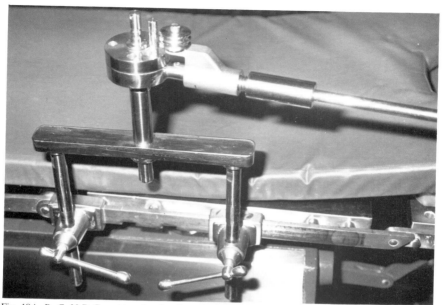

Fig. 10*A*, *B*, *C*. N.R.C. rod bender showing sequence of bending the rod.

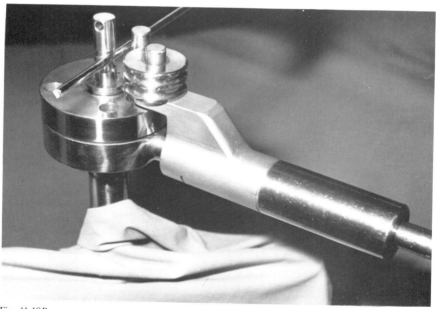

Fig. 11-10*B*.

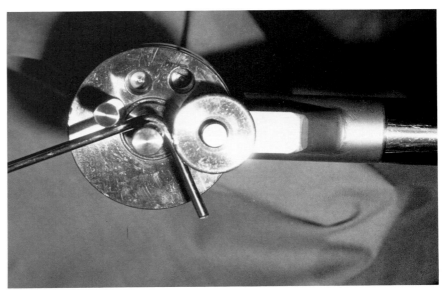

Fig. 11-10C.

Contouring and Bending Methods

The rod system has to be contoured carefully, not only to its laminar and sacral attachments but also to specifically maintain a normal lumbar lordosis (Fig. 11-9). Technically, this can prove difficult, especially when using 1/4-inch rods. A special bending tool was developed by the National Research Council of Canada, which has been very effective in reducing operating time and providing a consistently accurate means of bending (Fig. 11-10). It consists of two upright posts on a flat metal surface with a rotating arm containing a roller system, which minimizes surface damage to the rod.

Fusion

A posterolateral fusion is carried out down to the sacrum, with decortication of the sacral ala, and exposure and decortication of the transverse processes and pars interarticularis.

Pre- and Postoperative Management

Because this operation is in the category of high-risk surgery, careful neurologic assessment, including evaluation of bowel and bladder function, is mandatory. As previously stated, the assessment of the capacity of the sacral canal is very important, and if this is insufficient, an alternate method of attachment to the sacrum must be investigated.

Postoperatively, no immobilization is required, but again a careful assessment of the patient's neurologic status is required in the immediate postoperative phase.

Conclusions

The application of SSI to problems of the lumbosacral spine is not yet universally accepted. However, it is hoped that with improvements in the technique, it will find a place in the management of multiple-level disc degeneration in the unstable spine after wide laminectomy and in degenerative spondylolisthesis, as well as for stabilization of tumors.

There are several aspects to S.S.I. in the lumbar spine; first, in anything more than immobilizing above L2 lordosis should be introduced to avoid abnormal gait patterns. Secondly, crossing the sacro iliac joints, should be avoided whenever possible (Fig. 11-11). Thirdly, the use of rectangle or rhomboid bars to maintain length distraction and patency of the intervertebral foraminae is essential, and many mistakes in the past have originated from the use of double L rods (Fig. 11-12).

Another point of confusion is the rotatory characteristic of degenerative deformities. With normal S.S.I. technique the paravertebral bar lays at the base of the spinous processes. In these cases, the rods should lay as far forward as possible (close to the vertebral body in a lateral x-ray), over or in place of the facet aints and come to implant itself into the facet of S1 (Fig. 11-13).

This posterior lateral position corrects rotational deformities and avoids their recurrence.

The cephalad portion of the rectangle or rhomboid bars should always be bent into kyphosis and settled into a tunnel or through to avoid undue strains on the end wires.

Surprisingly enough, in our experience it has been more problematic to get an adequate fusion of a single joint, say L4-L5 than to fuse the entire lower back, e.g. L3-S1.

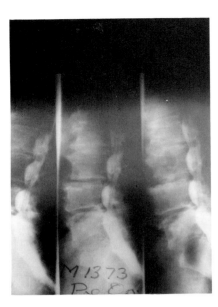

FIG. 11-11A. A 50 year old male with a retro-spondylolisthesis L4-L3, loss of lumbar lord-osis with a kyphosis L3-L2. Stenosis of the neural canal L3-L4, L4-L5. Osteoarthritis +4. Bulging discs L4-L5, L4-L3, L3-L2, L2-L1. Entrapped nerve root L3-L4.

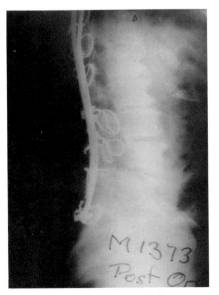

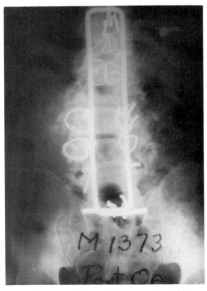

Figs. 11-11B & C. Total laminectoy S1-L2. For-aminectomy L3-L4. Reduction of kyphosis and retrospondylolisthesis, fixation under distrac-tion, rectangular configuration of rod, permits posterior stretching of intervertebral discs, creation of lordosis. S.S.I. fixation and posterio-lateral arthrodesis.

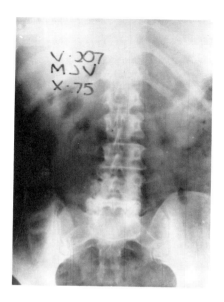

Figs. 11-12*A* & *B*. A 42 year old woman with a degenerative L4-S1 disc subluxated posterior facets at the same space with osteoarthritis. L5-S1 spondylolisthesis entrapped nerve root on the lateral recess of L4-L5.

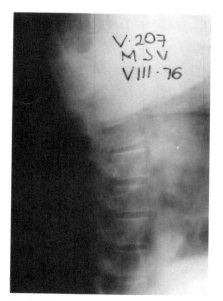

Fig. 11-12*B*.

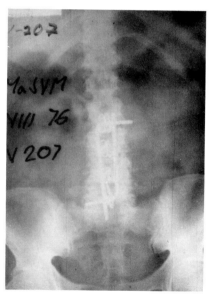

Figs. 11-12*C* & *D*. Correction by distraction and foraminectomy of the entrapped root at L4-L5. Fixation with double L rods S2-L2 with sublaminar wire. Posteriolateral arthrodesis.

Fig. 11-12*D*.

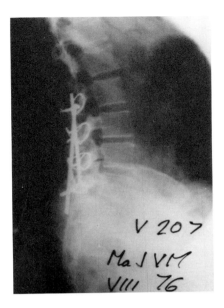

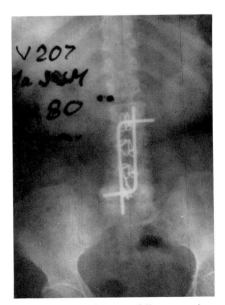

Figs. 11-12*E* & *F.* Four year follow up, patient asymptomatic, loss of correction L rod slipping, solid arthrodesis in situ.

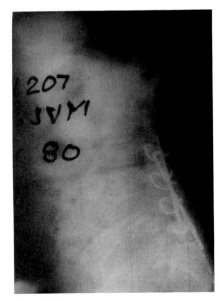

Fig. 11-12*F.*

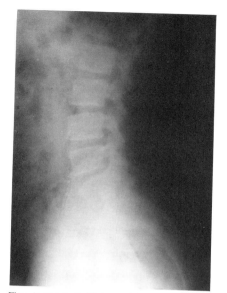 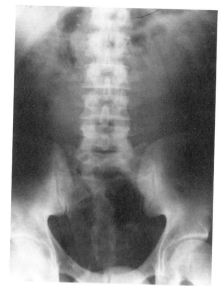

Figs. 11-13*A* & *B*. Male age 36 years with lumbarization, retrospondylolisthesis L4-L5 and degenerate I.V. disc at last movile segment.

Fig. 11-13*B*.

The correction and fixation of spondylolisthesis is still in question, but the real problem is whether the deformity merits correction and all the surgery that this might represent or simple arthrodesis in situ. If the deformity is incapacitating, our feeling, in that total or partial bony deformity removal is in order and then S.S.I. immobilization will act only as a scaffold to maintain length in a physiological position.

The most difficult deformities to reduce and maintain are kyphotic deformities of the lumbar spine, and total destruction of the osseous deformity is necessary in many of these cases (Fig. 11-14).

The question of fusing the herniated disc post removal is one that has intrigued many of us in the past and is still an unsolved question. Now evidence of indications are appearing with the long term results of quimolysis. As far as we are concerned a fusion is indicated in failed disc surgery, in unstable spines associated with herniated discs. In herniated discs with congenital osseous defects either at the sight of the herniation or adjacent to it.

Degenerative changes in the lumbar spine, which usually compose multiple pathologies at individual levels should be dealt with individually and each with its own merits and necessities, e.g. disc protrusions should be eliminated by anterior decompression hyperplastic yellow ligament by posterior decompression, osteoarthritis by posterior lateral fusion, neural canal stenosis by complete liberation, nerve entrapment syndromes by facet debridement and intervertebral foraminal enlargement, collapsing scoliosis by structural maintenance and arthrodesis, etc.

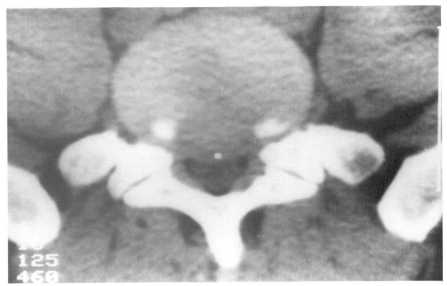

Figs. 11-13*C* & *D*. CAT scan showing spondylolisthesis and central protruded disc at last movile segment.

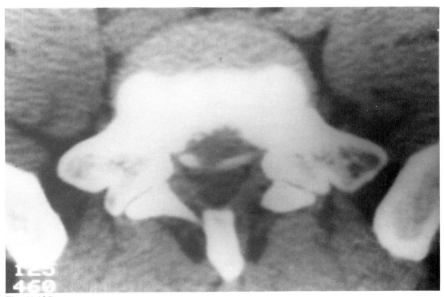

Fig. 11-13*D*.

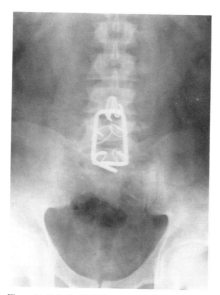

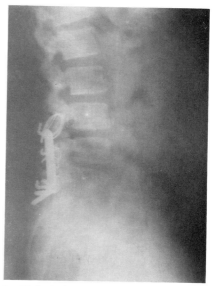

Figs. 11-13*E* & *F.* Discectomy, reduction of retrospondylolisthesis. Separation of posterior I.V. space fixation from S2-L4 with rhomboid bar. Notice it sits over the facet area and anterior to the lamina avoiding rotational stresses. Posteriolateral arthrodesis.

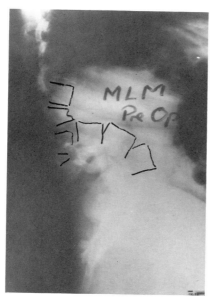

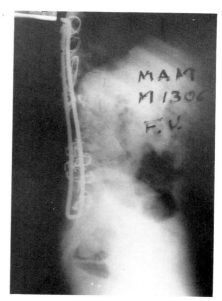

Figs. 11-14*A* & *B.* 26 year old woman with an acute 148° kyphosis in L3 paraparetic and getting worse congenital hemivertebra.

Fig. 11-14*B.*

Pathomechanics of Acute Thoracic and Lumbar Spinal Injuries

12

KELLY AND WHITESIDES HAVE POINTED out that in most circumstances, the front of the spine (vertebral bodies) is under compression while the back is under tension because the center of gravity is anterior to the spine.[7] Roaf was able to reproduce compression fractures experimentally by flexion, but he claimed never to have produced a concomitant rupture of the posterior ligaments.[11] Several contemporary authors have studied spinal flexion and reproduction of injuries in flexion. Among them, Panjabi has demonstrated that under flexion load, the thoracic spine functional unit was on the verge of instability when all ligaments posterior to and including the posterior half of the disk were cut.[10]

Nevertheless, in spite of an abundant amount of information on experimental spinal injuries resulting from flexion, there has not been much interest in the pattern of the instantaneous axis of flexion imposed by the testing machine in the determination of one particular type of fracture. There is no doubt that the flexion axis varies from case to case, but also in the same injury it changes with time. This variability in axis is related mainly to two different types of criteria:

1. *Intrinsic criteria:* The particular design and viscoelastic properties of the different parts of a spinal segment.

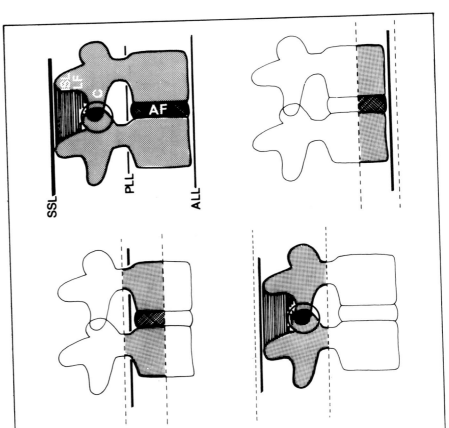

Fig. 12-1. The anterior column (*top right*), middle column (*bottom left*), and posterior column (*bottom right*) are illustrated. (From Denis F: The three column spine and its significance in the classification of acute thoracolumbar spinal injuries. Spine, 8:817-831, 1983.

2. *Extrinsic criteria:* How will the testing machine bend the spine? Will it, in other words, impose a specific mode of rotation of the sagittal plane around a fixed axis, or will it permit a variable axis?

Different loading rates and differing forces will also result in different fractures. The spine may be compared to a flexible beam. Whenever it is flexed, tension forces develop on the convex side and compression forces on the concave side. The axis of rotation is the neutral point which is not submitted to either compression or tension.

Depending upon the mode of flexion, the axis will vary. For instance, if an axial load is applied to the beam during flexion testing, the axis of flexion will displace toward the convexity of the bend, whereas the combination of axial load distraction and flexion testing will displace the axis of flexion toward the concavity.

This basic rule of physics applies also to the vertebral column and may assist the orthopedic surgeon in the comprehension of spinal injury mechanics.

Three-Column Spine Concept (Fig. 12-1)

In contrast to Holdsworth, who subdivided the spine into two columns and claimed that posterior ligamentous disruption alone produced instability, several experimental studies have demonstrated that instability or the ability to subluxate or dislocate appeared only after additional rupture of the posterior longitudinal ligament and of the annulus fibrosus.[2,5,8,10] Based on this evidence, the author has subdivided the spine into three columns.[3] The third column is represented by the structures that have to be torn in addition to Holdsworth's posterior ligamentous complex before the motion segment fails in flexion. The third column or middle column is, therefore, formed by the posterior half of the vertebral body, the posterior longitudinal ligament, and the posterior annulus fibrosus. The anterior column is composed of the anterior half of the vertebral body, the anterior longitudinal ligament, and the anterior half of the disk. Four different types of major spinal injuries can be identified on the basis of this concept: The compression fracture, the burst fracture, the seat-belt type injury, and fracture-dislocations.

Three-Flexion Axis Concept

This principal correlates well with the three-column spine concept in that flexion participates, to some degree, in more than 90% of spinal fractures. This may explain why the term "wedge fracture" (wastebasket diagnosis) has been used erroneously in describing major types of fractures, because all four types may present some anterior wedging of the vertebral body. Depending upon the instantaneous axis of flexion at the time of injury, a different type of fracture results.

1. When the axis is in the middle column, the posterior tension forces are comparable to the anterior compression forces. Depending upon the strength of bone and ligaments and the magnitude of the flexion force, a particular type of compression fracture will result. The middle column, acting as a hinge, will remain intact, preventing instability and injury of the neural elements (Figs. 12-2 and 12-3).

2. When the axis is in the anterior column close to the anterior longitudinal

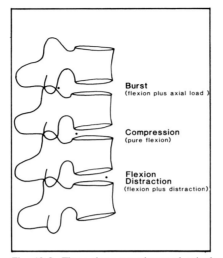

Fig. 12-2. These three superimposed spinal motion segments present three different instantaneous axes of flexion. The superior one has an axis in the posterior column, the middle one in the middle column, and the anterior one in the anterior column.

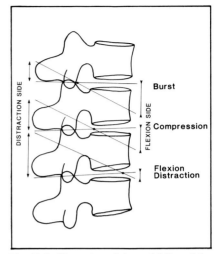

Fig. 12-3. Illustration of the variability of the anterior compression and posterior distraction moments depending upon the location of the instantaneous axis of flexion. The burst fracture has a posterior axis, which induces greater compression moments on the anterior and middle columns, whereas the anterior column alone is compressed in compression fractures, and both the posterior and middle columns are distracted in seat-belt type injuries (flexion-distraction).

ligament, the anterior compression force becomes minimal. On the contrary, posterior tension forces are great and will produce disruption of the posterior and middle columns (seat-belt type injuries).

3. The instantaneous axis of flexion may shift posteriorly when the axial load is combined with the flexion moment. When the axis is in the posterior column close to the posterior joints, the anterior compression component will become very large and will produce compression failure of both the anterior and the middle columns. The tension moment posteriorly is minimal, thus keeping the posterior ligamentous complex intact. The posterior half of the vertebral body's anterior shield of the neural elements is retropulsed into the spinal canal, leading to neurologic damage in 50% of the cases. Smith and Kaufer have described this as hyperflexion, and others have termed it flexion-distraction.[12] These are basically the seat-belt type injuries (Fig. 12-3).

4. The instantaneous axis of flexion may be shifted laterally away from the spinal column by rotation, leading to a fracture-dislocation of the flexion-rotation type (three-column rupture). If the flexion axis is anterior to the spine, the flexion moment induces mainly distraction, accounting for the flexion-distraction fracture-dislocation. Rarely, the flexion is reversed into extension in what has been traditionally called "shear injuries." In that situation, the instantaneous axis of exten-

sion may be in the middle column, which places the anterior longitudinal ligament under tension and the posterior facets under compression. When the extension axis reaches the posterior column, or even extends posterior to it, the force extending the spine may become large enough to rupture sequentially the anterior longitudinal ligament, and disk, the posterior longitudinal ligament, and even the ligamentum flavum and interspinous ligament as all those structures are submitted to the anterior tension force. If the force is even greater, it may shear off one segment of the spine, breaking the posterior arch off as the superior segment is displaced anteriorly, leading to the typical shear injury.

Anatomic-Clinical Correlation in the Presence of a Neurologic Deficit in Spinal Trauma

A causal relationship between the neural deficit and the type of fracture is accepted by some and denied by many. However, there simply has to be a reason why the cord or cauda equina has been damaged. The neural structure either has been hit, cut compressed, distracted, or affected in some other way. The phenomenon of spinal cord injuries without radiographic abnormalities in children illustrates the problem very well.[9] Fifty-two percent of these children present with a delayed paralysis up to four days after injury. Most of them recalled transient paresthesia, numbness, or subjective paralysis. The possibility of a cord injury with a closed and intact spinal canal has been raised by some. It could then be related to either an overdistraction of the cord or to a concussion of the cord by the posterior arch. This would occur when a direct blow is applied to the back without any deformation of the canal (even temporarily) in a manner similar to the mechanism of brain damage in closed head injuries without skull fracture.

The other possible cord concussion mechanism that shows no radiographic changes may be explained by unrecognized reduced fracture-dislocations and posterior arch fractures that have momentarily crushed the cord in a direct blow to the spine. This latter etiology is more frequent in children, perhaps because their posterior arches are shorter, weaker, and poorly protected by the thin soft-tissue layer that covers the posterior arch in the back. Bazilevskaia recently analyzed 128 patients who had died after trauma to the cervical and thoracic spine and spinal cord.[1] In all cases, the vertebral canal was damaged, demonstrating a direct mechanical injury of the neural structures. In 85% of the cases, there was evidence of fractures with or without subluxation. In the 15% remaining, there was evidence of severe ligamentous disruptions, although there was no displacement.

The three-column system corroborates these postmortem findings in a series of 412 spinal injuries studied by the author, with 197 cases of *compression fractures* without neurologic injuries other than related to associated problems (cervical spine fracture-dislocations or severe Malgaigne pelvic injury).[3] This tended to confirm the fact that an intact spinal neural canal is good protection for the neural

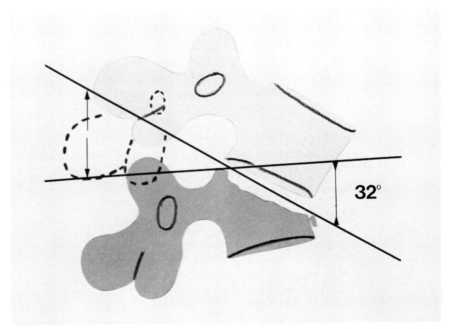

Fig. 12-4A. The increase in intertransverse distance is 2.5 times greater (20 mm instead of 8 mm) in the seat-belt type injury (*right*) than in the compression fracture (*left*), even for a lesser amount of flexion (27 degrees instead of 32 degrees).

structures. *Burst fractures* were associated with neurologic deficits in 50% of patients, all with bone penetration into the canal. *Seat-belt type injuries* were not associated with neurologic problems, perhaps because they were lumbar (in front of the cauda equina) and because particular attention was given to identifying flexion-distraction fracture-dislocations as a separate entity caused by a similar mechanism but with greater energy expenditure. *Fracture-dislocations,* in 75% of the cases, presented with neurologic deficits (about half of which were complete paraplegias), all of them with significant disruptions of the spinal canal's continuity.

Classification of Major Thoracic and Lumbar Spinal Injuries

Compression Fractures

Biomechanics: The compression fracture results from a flexion force, the instantaneous axis of which is situated in the middle column. This flexion force

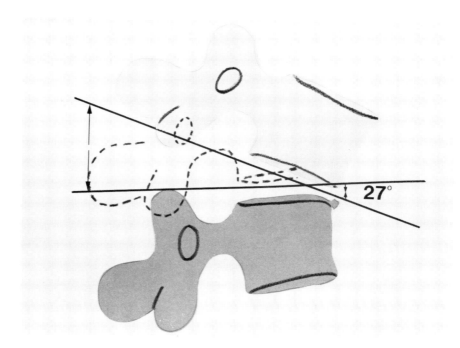

Fig. 12-4*B*.

results in compression failure of the anterior column. The middle column is acting as a hinge, thus remaining in a neutral zone between compression and tension forces. It is intact in terms of the posterior wall of the vertebral body. The posterior column may be partially disrupted depending upon the amount of anterior collapse at the point of maximal deformation. The different ligaments of the posterior complex rupture in a sequence, starting posteriorly and moving anteriorly all the way to the ligamentum flavum. The explanation for this is based on the greater deformation—the further away from the axis, the greater the tension. The posterior interspinous ligaments may be stretched two centimeters when the ligamentum flavum is stretched only one. The transverse processes will rarely be split horizontally by the pull of the intertransverse membrane because the increase in the intertransverse distance is seldom comparable to that occurring in a seat-belt type injury (Fig. 12-4). The spinous process and lamina are frequently avulsed by the stronger ligaments, producing a horizontal fracture.

Subtypes: The two main subtypes of compression fractures are anterior and lateral compression fractures, related respectively to anterior flexion and lateral flexion (Fig. 12-5). It should be noted that the part of the vertebral body that gives way may be isolated to the superior end-plate, the inferior end-plate, both of them, or the midpart of the vertebra between them (Fig. 12-6). This is not very significant but may dictate which interspinous ligament will be disrupted; the superior inter-

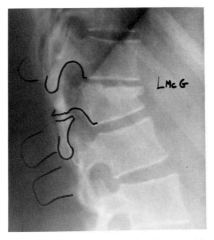

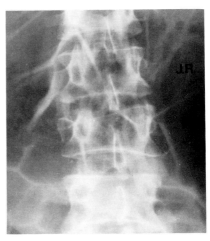

Fig. 12-5A. Anterior compression fracture with disruption of the superior end-plate (Type B compression fracture). Note the normal height of the posterior part of the vertebral body. The interspinous ligament was torn and the pars interarticularis fractured. These findings are frequent when the loss of height of the anterior vertebral body is greater than 50%.

B, Lateral compression fracture. (From Denis F: The three column spine and its significance in the classification of acute thoracolumbar spinal injuries. Spine, 8:817-831, 1983.

spinous ligament if the superior end-plate is crushed, and the inferior interspinous ligament when the inferior end-plate is damaged.

Roentgenographic Characteristics of Compression Fractures: On the lateral roentgenogram as well as on the CAT scan, one may verify the intactness of the posterior wall and its good alignment with the adjacent vertebral bodies (Fig. 12-7).

Burst Fractures

Biomechanics: The major component of stress on the vertebra is axial load. When some flexion is present, the instantaneous axis of flexion is within the posterior column or even further behind it (Fig. 12-3). Although axial load represents the greater component of the mechanism, it may be combined with other forces, in particular, flexion (anterior or lateral) and even rotation. The fact that the flexion hinge is posterior minimizes the tension forces on the posterior ligamentous complex, but maximizes the compression stress on the anterior and middle columns, leading to a failure under compression of the whole vertebral body including the posterior wall. The sequence of events is as follows: (1) build-up of intradiscal pressure, (2) end-plate load, (3) end-plate deformation, (4) end-plate failure, penetration of the disk into the vertebral body, and build-up of pressure inside it, and (5) explosion with splaying of the fragments of end-plate, concomitant splaying of the posterior arch (which may fracture at the level of the

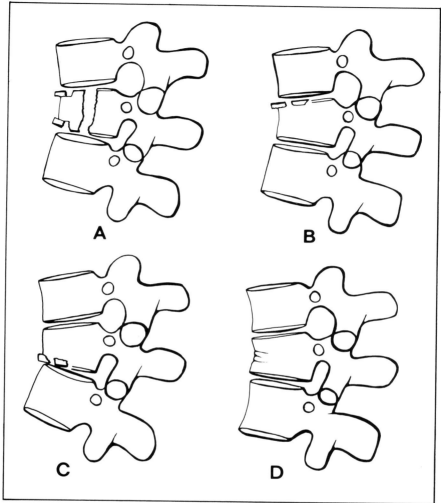

Fig. 12-6. Subclassification of compression fractures. (From Denis F: The three column spine and its significance in the classification of acute thoracolumbar spinal injuries. Spine, 8:817-831, 1983.

anterior cortex of the lamina as it opens like a wishbone), and retropulsion of the posterocentral fragment of the end-plate into the spinal canal. This fragment remains attached to the annulus fibrosus and, therefore, rotates upward (superior end-plate) as it is retropulsed. The posterocentral end-plate fragment macroscopically is usually in one or two pieces (sagittal split of the two pieces), and the angle between its superior end-plate side and its posterior wall side is more acute than in a normal vertebra. The implication is that the angle was closed by compression before it was fractured and displaced backward.

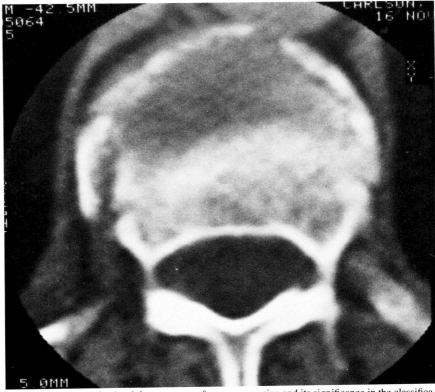

Fig. 12-7. Computerized axial tomogram of compression fracture. Note anterior end-plate fracture and totally intact posterior wall of the vertebral body. (From Denis F: The three column spine and its significance in the classification of acute thoracolumbar spinal injuries. Spine, 8:817-831, 1983.

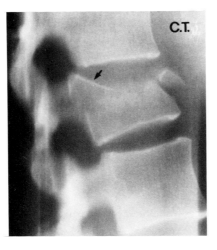

Fig. 12-8. Lateral tomogram of a burst fracture (Type B). Note
—Severe disruption of superior end-plate
—Loss of height of posterior vertebral body
—Fracture of posterior wall of body.

The arrow shows the large fragment retropulsed into the canal. (From Denis F: The three column spine and its significance in the classification of acute thoracolumbar spinal injuries. Spine, 8:817-831, 1983.

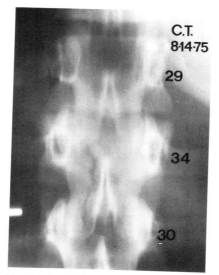 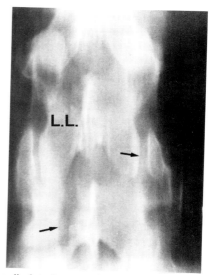

Fig. 12-9A and B. Anteroposterior tomogram of two burst fractures. Note the increased inter-pediculate distances, the vertical laminar fractures, and the splayed facet joints.

Finally, there is an implosion. Kazarian has demonstrated that following the burst (explosion), the vertebra does not remain in the position of maximal displacement.[6] This is related to the ligamentous network that keeps the vertebrae together as well as to the viscoelastic properties of the vertebral body. It is quite likely that the pressure remaining over the neural elements at the time of examination is less than at the time of maximal deformation. The increase in interpediculate distance, the measurable index of posterior arch splaying, does not return quite to normal after explosion but still decreases significantly, locking the fragment of bone inside the spinal canal.

Roentgenographic Characteristics: The compression failure of the middle column is suggested on the lateral film by the displaced fracture of the cortex of the posterior wall, and by tilting and retropulsion of the fragment of bone into the spinal canal (Fig. 12-8). The fragment may come from either end-plate or from both. On an anteroposterior roentgenogram, one may recognize the pathognomonic increase in the interpediculate distance, the vertical fracture of the lamina, and the accompanying splaying of the posterior facets. All three signs corroborate the splaying of the entire posterior arch at the interpediculate level (Fig. 12-9).

CAT Scan Characteristics: The vertebral ring, which was intact in compression fractures, is ruptured in two places: the posterior wall and the lamina. The break in the posterior wall is accompanied by retropulsion of a large fragment back into the canal against the neural elements (Fig. 12-10).

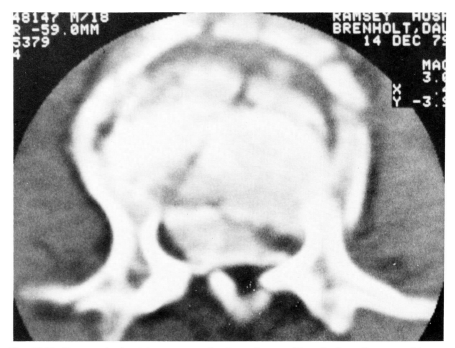

Fig. 12-10. Computerized axial tomogram of a burst fracture. Note the large fragment of bone retropulsed from the posterior wall.

Types of Burst Fractures (Fig. 12-11)

Type A: Both end-plates have burst, and both have retropulsed a fragment into the neural canal (Fig. 12-12). This fracture results from pure axial load and is mainly encountered in the low lumbar spine.

Type B: This is characterized by burst of the superior end-plate, with frequent midline sagittal fracture of the inferior end-plate and participation of the lower end-plate in the splaying of the body. The latter does not retropulse bone at the lower level into the canal. It is the most frequent burst fracture and results from a combination of flexion and axial load. The thoracolumbar junction (T12, L1, L2) is the most frequent location of this type of fracture (Figs. 12-3 and 12-14).

Type C: Burst of the inferior end-plate is rare and has not been encountered yet with neurologic damage. It results also from the axial load and flexion (Fig. 12-15).

Type D: Burst rotation appears typically in the midlumbar spine and looks like a fracture-dislocation because of its rotational component. It presents all the signs of a burst fracture, however: The vertebral body is comminuted, the interpediculate distance is increased, the lamina is fractured vertically, and the lateral film does not show any subluxation or dislocation but confirms the presence of bone retropulsed

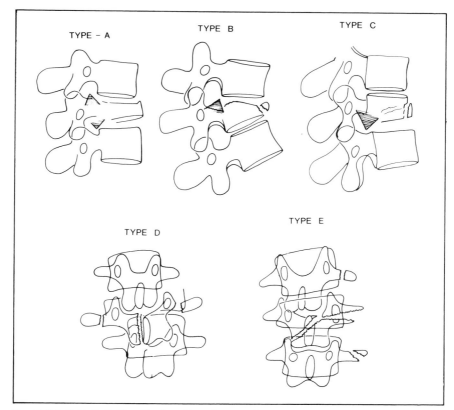

Fig. 12-11*A, B, C, D, E.* Classification of burst fractures: Types A, B, and C are mainly diagnosed from the lateral roentgenogram. Their anteroposterior roentgenograms reveal the basic pathognomonic features seen in Fig. 12-8. Types D and E are diagnosed from anteroposterior roentgenograms. The lateral film of a Type D looks like a Type A, whereas the lateral film of a Type E may look like Type A, B, or C. (From Denis F: The three column spine and its significance in the classification of acute thoracolumbar spinal injuries. Spine, 8:817-831, 1983.

into the spinal canal. Both myelograms and CAT scans demonstrate that the obstruction is due to bone retropulsion and not to offset, as in fracture-dislocations (Fig. 12-16).

Type E: Burst lateral flexion presents with a wedge on anteroposterior roentgenography, increase of the interpediculate distance, and an oblique laminar fracture, sometimes with splitting of one transverse process and pedicle horizontally (demonstration of the tension forces on that side). The lateral flexion component of the fracture may also be expressed by an ipsilateral avulsion fracture of the lumbar transverse processes. The lateral burst fracture is significantly different from the lateral compression fracture in that there is bone in the canal and neurologic damage is frequent (Fig. 12-17).

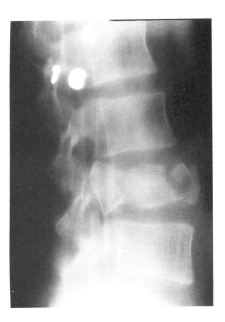

Fig. 12-12. Type A burst fracture.

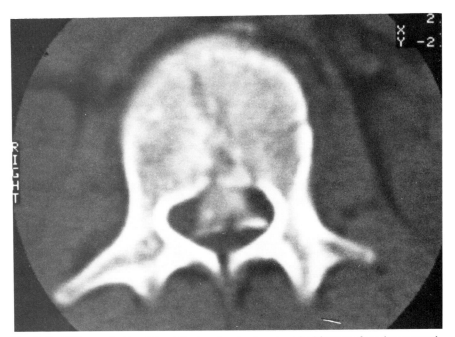

Fig. 12-13. CAT scan of a Type B burst fracture showing the retropulsed fragment from the upper end-plate and the sagittal split of the lower end-plate.

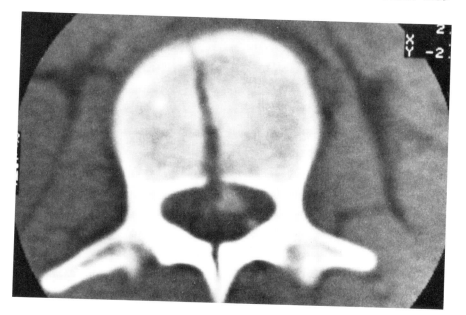

Seat-Belt Type Injury

Biomechanics: Flexion-distraction is the mechanism of seat-belt type injuries. The axis of flexion is in the anterior column, making the anterior annulus fibrosus the hinge of flexion. The posterior tension forces rupture both the posterior and middle columns through ligaments or bone or a combination thereof. The minimal compression anteriorly may produce a "mini-compression fracture" involving about five to ten percent of the height of the anterior body. It should not be confused with a flexion-distraction fracture-dislocation, since the latter presents frequently with significant neural damage, which is rare in the former. An intriguing question about seat-belt type injuries is the mechanism leading to the usual horizontal split of the transverse process and pedicle. The author's hypothesis about this mechanism is based on the increase in tension in the intertransverse membrane due to a significant increase in the intertransverse distance in seat-belt type injuries as compared with compression fractures. The same amount of flexion (same angle) will increase the intertransverse distance more significantly when the axis of flexion is anterior (Fig. 12-18).

Roentgenographic Characteristics: An increase in the interspinous distance, horizontal split of transverse processes and pedicles, pars interarticularis fractures, increased height of the posterior vertebral body, horizontal fractures through the vertebral body (Chance fracture), and posterior opening of the disk space (ligamentous rupture of the middle column) can be seen on roentgenographic examination. Computerized axial tomography is not particularly useful in this type of injury

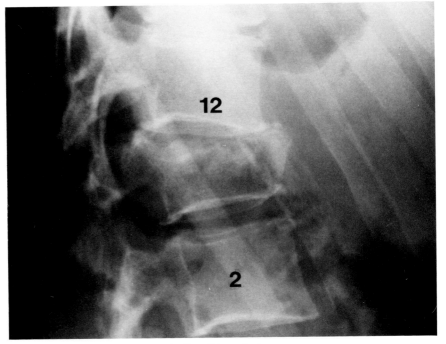

Fig. 12-14*A*. Lateral roentgenogram of a Type B burst fracture.

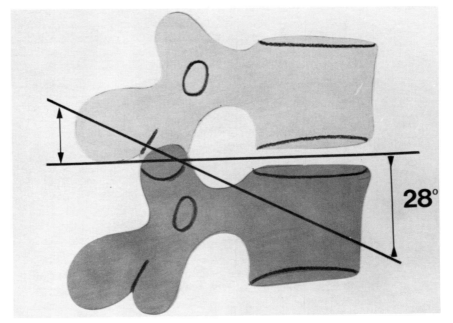

Fig. 12-14*B*.

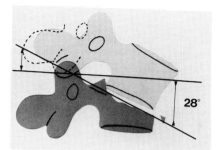

Fig. 12-14C.

28°

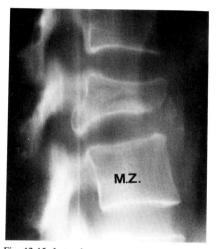

M.Z.

Fig. 12-15. Lateral roentgenogram of a Type C burst fracture.

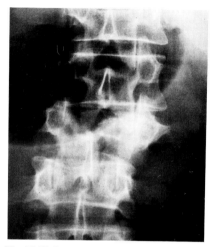

Fig. 12-16. Lateral roentgenogram of a Type D burst fracture.

because it is only through sagittal reconstruction that one can identify the fracture. The quality of detail and definition obtained by sagittal reconstruction is usually inferior to that of a lateral tomogram.

Subtypes of Seat-Belt Injuries: Seat-belt injuries may involve one or two levels. The injury may be mainly ligamentous or bony. This differentiation, although seemingly unnecessary, may help in therapeutic decisions, since it is a proven fact that ligaments do not heal as well as bone (Fig. 12-19).

Fracture Dislocations

Biomechanics: In fracture-dislocations, all three columns are significantly damaged by different combinations of forces. The mechanisms of failure are mainly flexion-rotation, rotation, shear, and flexion-distraction.

General Roentgenographic Characteristics: Most important is the evidence of

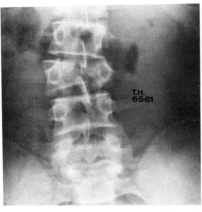

Fig. 12-17. Lateral roentgenogram of a Type E burst fracture.

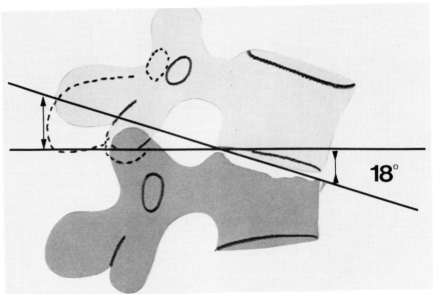

Fig. 12-18A. Demonstration of significant increase in intertransverse distance in the Chance fracture as compared with a compression fracture of similar angulation.

subluxation or dislocation on anteroposterior or lateral x-rays. Other frequent signs are multiple rib fractures, multiple transverse process fractures, unilateral articular process fractures, horizontal laminar fractures, and spinous process fractures. Computerized axial tomography will demonstrate the offset of the spinal canal and the resulting obstruction (Fig. 12-20)

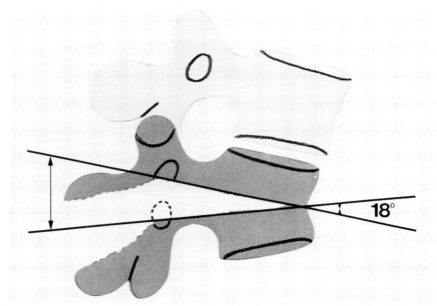

Fig. 12-18*B*.

Flexion-Rotation Fracture-Dislocations: There is a spectrum of injuries involving both flexion and rotation, with different quantities of both forces. One could actually say that the flexion-rotation fracture-dislocation is the central part of a spectrum that starts on one end with flexion-distraction and ends on the other with pure rotation. The anterior and middle columns may fail under a combination of compression and rotation through bone (slice fracture) or under rotation alone (through disk) (Fig. 12-21). The pathognomonic sign of flexion-rotation is the rotational failure of the superior articular process of the inferior vertebra, which is sheared off by the inferior articular process of the vertebra above. The posterior column is also ruptured under tension (induced by flexion), leading to what Holdsworth has interpreted as the definite sign of instability of the posterior ligamentous complex. Although true in fracture-dislocations, it may occur also in the three other major types of spinal injuries with a variable significance in terms of stability. As a matter of fact, pure rotational fracture-dislocations are frequently seen in the upper thoracic spine (T3-T4 or T4-T5) with an intact supraspinous and interspinous ligament when everything else has been disrupted in front of those two structures. The anterolateral periosteum and the anterior longitudinal ligament may be more-or-less damaged. They tend to be relatively intact in slice fracture-dislocations, whereas they will be more disrupted in pure rotational dislocations. *Shear Fracture-Dislocations:* All three columns are disrupted starting with the anterior longitudinal ligament because these injuries start in extension, inducing tension forces on the anterior column and compression forces on the posterior

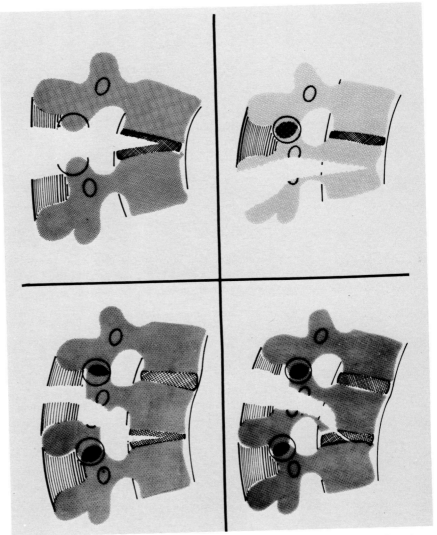

Fig. 12-19. One level seat-belt type injury through bone (Chance fracture) (*top right*). One level seat-belt type injury through the ligaments (*top left*). Two level seat-belt type injury through bone at the level of the middle column (*bottom right*). Two level seat-belt type injury through ligaments at the level of the middle column (*bottom left*). (From Denis F: The three column spine and its significance in the classification of acute thoracolumbar spinal injuries. Spine, 8:817-831, 1983.

column (Fig. 12-22). The continued shearing force dislocates one segment of the spine in front of the other. A typical mechanism is a powerful blow to the back (five out of nine patients seen by the author were lumberjacks who were hit across the back by somebody else's falling tree.)

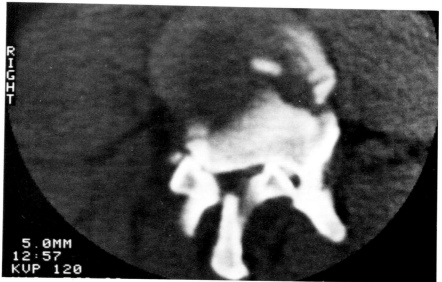

Fig. 12-20. Computerized axial tomogram of an L2-L3 lumbar fracture-dislocation of the flexion-rotation type through the disk. Note the fracture of the left superior articular process (*top right*). (From Denis F: The three column spine and its significance in the classification of acute thoracolumbar spinal injuries. Spine, 8:817-831, 1983.

There are two possible subtypes of shear fracture-dislocations. The most frequent is the posteroanterior subtype, the other is the anteroposterior form. In the posteroanterior shear subtype, the segment above shears off in front of the segment below (Fig. 12-23). This takes place in the extended position so that the vertebral bodies are intact without any loss of anterior or posterior height. On the contrary, the posterior arch of the dislocating vertebral segment is fractured at several levels owing to its difficulties in clearing the posterior arch at the level below and also to the compression force applied to the posterior arch by the extension moment. As a result of this, the posterior approach will often disclose a free-floating lamina, fractures of several spinous processes in the upper segment, and fracture of the superior facet of the lower vertebra (different from the superior articular process fracture seen in flexion-rotation injuries). Complete rupture of the anterior longitudinal ligament is demonstrated by operative observation or accidental over-distraction obtained when distraction instrumentation alone is used. Complete disruption of the spinal cord and dural leak occur.

Characteristics of the Anteroposterior Shear: In this particular subtype, the segment above shears away from the segment below in a posterior direction (Fig. 12-24). The posterior arch of the segment above has nothing to clear in its posterior displacement. The posterior translation of the upper segment also minimizes the compression forces applied to the posterior arch by the extension moment. There may be, however, a fracture of the spinous process.

Fracture-Dislocation of the Flexion-Distraction Type: This resembles the seat-belt

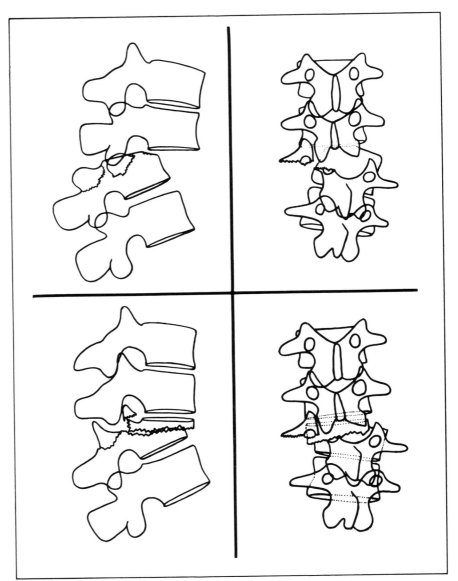

Fig. 12-21. Lateral diagram of a fracture-dislocation of the flexion-rotation type through bone (slice fracture) (*bottom left*). Anteroposterior diagram of a fracture-dislocation of the flexion-rotation type through bone (slice fracture). Note the difference in rotation between both spinal segments (*bottom right*). Lateral diagram of a fracture-dislocation of the flexion-rotation type through the disk. Note the superior articular process fracture on one side only (*top left*). Anteroposterior diagram of a fracture-dislocation of the flexion-rotation type through the disk. Note the fracture of the left superior articular process (*top right*). (From Denis: The three column spine and its significance in the classification of acute thoracolumbar spinal injuries. Spine, 8:817-831, 1983)

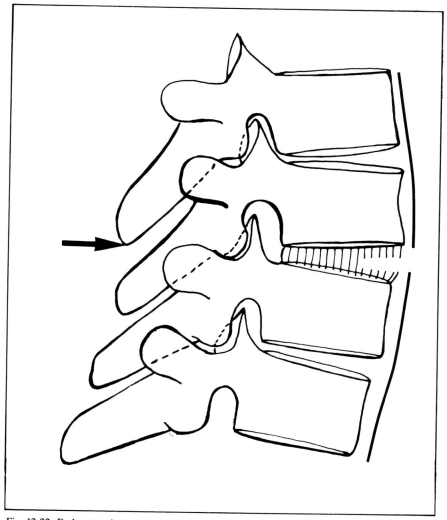

Fig. 12-22. Early extension moment, which is involved in the disruption of the anterior longitudinal ligament.

type injury, which included rupture of both the posterior and middle columns under tension. In this case, the entire annulus fibrosus is torn, allowing the vertebra above to subluxate or dislocate on the vertebra below. This is accompanied by stripping of the anterior longitudinal ligament of the lower vertebra without necessarily disrupting its continuity. On roentgenography, it presents all the characteristics of the seatbelt type injury, with a split of the transverse processes and pedicles bilaterally. In addition, the lateral film shows subluxation or dislocation (Fig. 12-25).

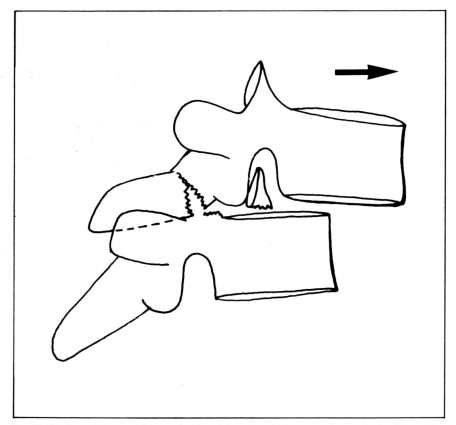

Fig. 12-23A. Lateral diagram of a posterior shear injury. Note the intact anterior vertebral bodies and the fracture of the superior articular facet, which has been sheared off by the anterior displacement. The spinous process or entire posterior arch may be fractured by the same mechanism. (From Denis F: The three column spine and its significance in the classification of acute thoracolumbar spinal injuries. Spine, 8:817-831, 1983

Editor's Commentary

There are several important observations and questions concerning the pathology of spine injuries. We often consider the compression fracture of the thoracic and lumbar spine that is no more than 30% involved as automatically not

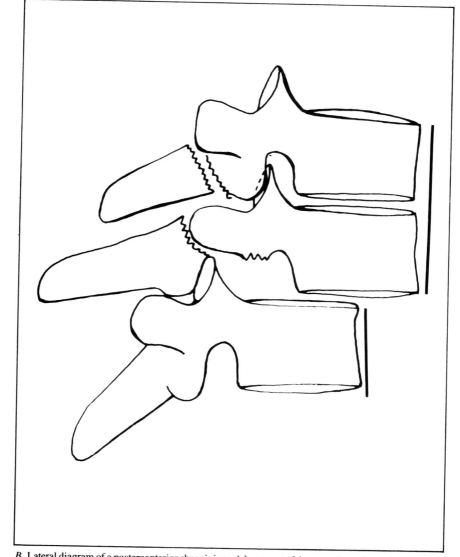

B, Lateral diagram of a posteroanterior shear injury. A large part of the posterior arch may be left behind (floating lamina). (From Denis F: The three column spine and its significance in the classification of acute thoracolumbar spinal injuries. Spine, 8:817-831, 1983)

surgically correctable. Yet in my personal practice, the postoperative follow-up of old cases after ten years or more revealed progressive deformity (1) during the acute stage due to recognized comminution, (2) by degeneration due to a recognized disc

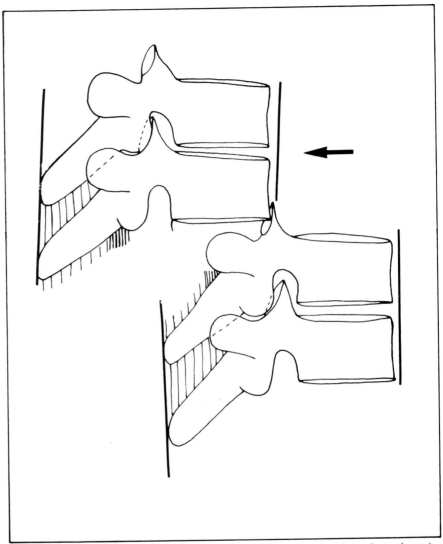

Fig. 12-24A. Lateral diagram of an anteroposterior shear injury. The posterior arches and anterior vertebral bodies may be entirely intact, but the three ligamentous columns are disrupted. (From Denis F: The three column spine and its significance in the classification of acute thoracolumbar spinal injuries. Spine, 8:817-831, 1983

lesion in conjunction with the fracture, and (3) in the form of osteoarthritic facet changes and pain (Fig. 12-26).

As in other kyphotic deformities, bone plasticity and settling with age are, no doubt, associated with a progressive deformity with invalidating pathologic

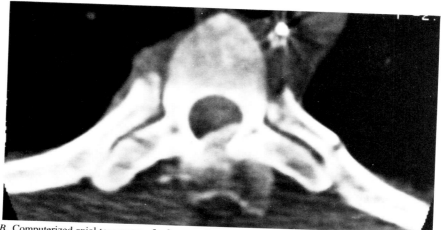

B, Computerized axial tomogram of a fracture-dislocation of the anteroposterior shear type. Note the anterior aspect of the superior vertebral body locked on the superior facets of the inferior vertebral body. (From Denis F: The three column spine and its significance in the classification of acute thoracolumbar spinal injuries. Spine, 8:817-831, 1983

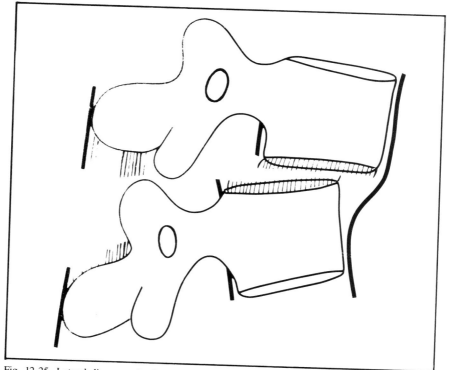

Fig. 12-25. Lateral diagram of a fracture-dislocation of the flexion-distraction type. The posterior, middle, and anterior ligamentous columns are disrupted but for the anterior longitudinal ligament which strips off the vertebral body below. (From Denis F: The three column spine and its significance in the classification of acute thoracolumbar spinal injuries. Spine, 8:817-831, 1983

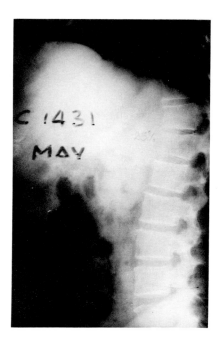

Fig. 12-26A. A 30-year-old male with a T12 compression fracture with 25% involvement. Treatment was bed rest, Jewett brace, and analgesics.

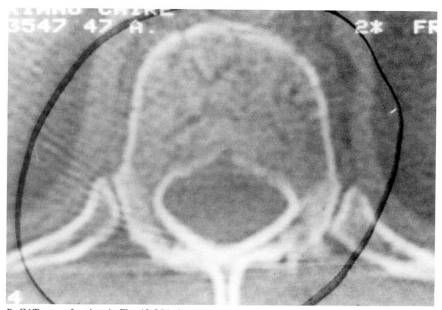

B, CAT scan of patient in Fig. 12-26A shows comminuted fracture of the T12 vertebral body.

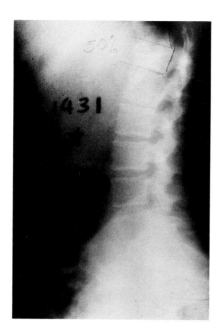

C, Same patient as in Fig. 12-26*A*, two months later, with a 50% compression fracture in spite of external support.

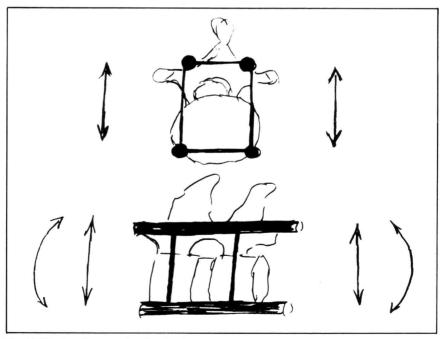

Fig. 12-27. Anterior-posterior fixation for the unstable fracture-dislocation to reduce rotational instability should be considered, as it is for other spine deformities.

changes. What is not clear is when and how much treatment should be given in the future to these seemingly inconsequential lesions.

Instability of a fractured spine should be considered any deformity that involves more than one column, eg, posterior and middle column, anterior and middle column, or all three columns. Burst fractures, on the other hand, are all characterized by bone protrusion into the neural canal. Only ± 50% have neurologic symptomatology. Again the question arises, for those without neurologic involvement, should anterior decompression of the canal be done, should nothing be done, or should a localized arthrodesis at the pathologic site be done? There is no record in the literature elucidating the ultimate fate of these individuals. Yet we occasionally see one totally healed with increasing discomfort and neurologic signs.

Fracture-dislocations have, as mentioned in this chapter, a rotational instability. To correct and maintain such a deformity, posterior instrumentation is characteristically inadequate. Several anterior fixating devices are now available: Gardner, Bradford, and Dunn, for example. However, they also have poor fixation. Up until now, nobody has considered anterior-posterior instrumentation for this condition (Fig. 12-27).

Neurologic salvage is directly proportional to neural canal alignment and decompression. What is too much surgery?

Finally, we have thought of paraplegics as "sitters," even though from the clinical history and type of lesion we can pretty well anticipate the prognosis.[13] Our treatment, a complete fusion of the spine to relieve pressure on the ischial tuberosities and sacrum on sitting and to decrease energy expenditure during transference procedures, has now been reinforced by the reciprocal swivel walker. This device automatically makes walkers out of these patients, who were previously condemned to a wheelchair.

References

1. Bazilevskaia Z: State of Vertebral Canal in Vertebral and Cord Injuries: Zh-Vopr-Neirokhir (4)54-59, July-August 1978.

2. Bedbrook GM: Spinal injuries with tetraplegia and paraplegia. J Bone Jt Surg 61B:267-284, 1979.

3. Denis F: The three column spine and its significance in the classification of acute thoracolumbar spinal injuries. Spine (*in press*).

4. Denis F, Armstrong GWD: Burst fractures in the lumbar spine. Ortho Trans 5:417, 1981.

5. Holdsworth FW: Fractures, dislocations, and fracture-dislocation of the spine. J Bone Jt Surg 52A:1534-1551, 1970.

6. Kazarian L, Graves GA: Comprehensive strength characteristics of human vertebral centrum. Spine 2:1-14, 1977.

7. Kelly RP, Whitesides TE Jr: Treatment of lumbodorsal fracture dislocations. Ann Surg 167:705, 1968.

8. Nagel DA, Koogle TA, Piziali RL, Perkash I: Stability of the upper lumbar spine following progressive disruption and the application of individual internal and external fixation devices. J Bone Jt Surg 63A:62-70, 1981.

9. Pang D, Wilberger JE: Spinal cord injury without radiographic abnormalities in children. J Neurosurg 57:114-129, 1982.

10. Panjabi MM, Hausfeld JN, White AA: A biomechanic study of the ligamentous stability of the thoracic spine. Acta Ortho Scand 52:315-326, 1981.

11. Roaf R: A study of the mechanics of spinal injuries. J Bone Jt Surg 42B:810-823, 1960.

12. Smith WS, Kaufer H: Patterns and mechanisms of lumbar injuries associated with lap seat belts. J Bone Jt Surg 51A:239-254, 1969.

13. Rose GK: The principles and practice of hip guidance articulations. Prosthetics Orthotics Inter 3:37-43, 1979.

Fractures of the Thoracolumbar Spine Treated with SSI

13

Introduction

The principles for treating fractures of the spine with SSI are:

1. Correction of the deformity by using the bars as lever arms.

2. Rigid internal fixation to maintain the correction without using external immobilization postoperatively.

In our work, we previously followed the classic principles of the two-column theory for the classification of fractures, but at present we employ the three-column theory of Denis.

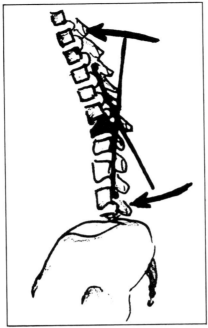

Fig. 13-1. Second-degree lever arm is applied with the bars for correction of kyphotic deformities.

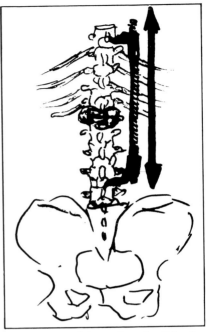

Fig. 13-2. Use of the outrigger for distraction and reduction in severe compression and burst fractures.

Management

Initial treatment for these patients after the injury includes the following:

1. Complete history and physical examination to determine the general status of the patient and the neurologic status for prognostic purposes.

2. Radiologic examination to classify the fracture. This includes simple radiographs, tomograms, myelograms, and CAT scans.

The cardiovascular, pulmonary, urinary, and dermatologic systems are stabilized prior to surgical treatment. Only cases with a progressive neurologic deficit are considered an emergency in need of immediate surgery.

All patients are placed on Stryker frames or CircOLectric beds before surgery.

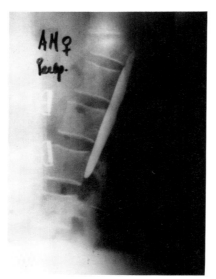

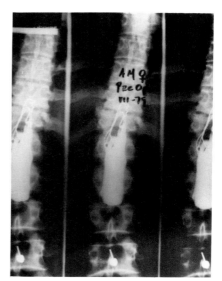

Fig. 13-3. Twenty-four-year-old female with fracture-dislocation of T11 and T12 due to a car accident, with resultant complete paraplegia. *A* and *B*, Preoperative myelograms. *C* and *D*, Postoperative x-rays.

Fig. 13-3*B*.

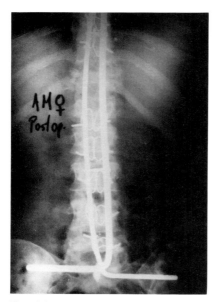

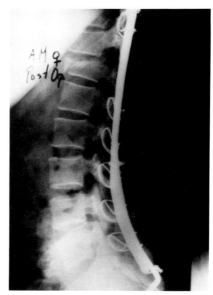

Fig. 13-3*C*.

Fig. 13-3*D*.

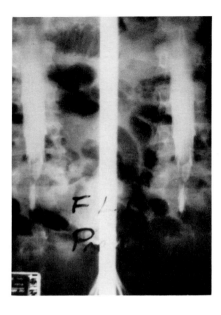

Fig. 13-4. Twenty-nine-year-old male who was thrown out of a car. He has a fracture-dislocation of L5-S1. Intense lumbosacral pain radiates down the left leg, which was paretic and hyporeflexive. *A* and *B*, Preoperative myelogram. *C* and *D*, Postoperative results with 100% reduction. Complete neurologic recovery was obtained.

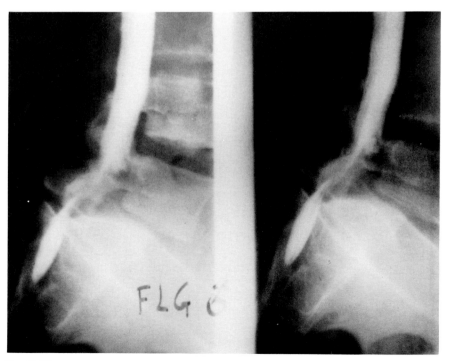

Fig. 13-4*B*.

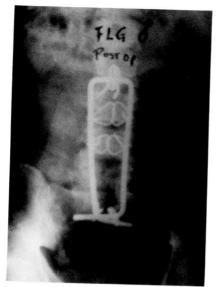

Fig. 13-4C.

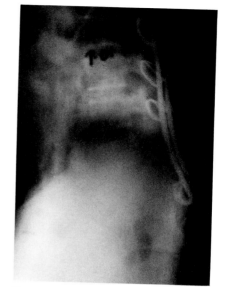

Fig. 13-4D.

Surgical Procedure

The routine posterior approach to the spine is used in the affected region, followed by reduction of the fracture and the spinal canal. Fixation with SSI is then done.

Reduction of the obstruction of the spinal canal is achieved through laminectomy, diskectomy, corpectomy, or combinations thereof. In the difficult burst fracture, in which the posterior wall of the vertebral body or the disk, or both, retropulsed into the spinal canal, we choose the method used by Henning, which consists of decancellation of the body through the pedicle (Fig. 13-6). This decreases the amount of bleeding considerably and protects the spinal canal from further injury. The retropulsed fragments are tapped back into place after decancellation (Fig. 13-6D).

The fracture-dislocation is treated with laminectomy and facetectomy to reduce the canal (Figs. 13-4 and 13-5), and in SSI the two bars acting as second-degree lever arms are used to reduce excessive kyphosis or lateral deviation (Fig. 13-1). To reestablish length, an outrigger is used when an intact longitudinal ligament is present (burst fractures) (Fig. 13-2).

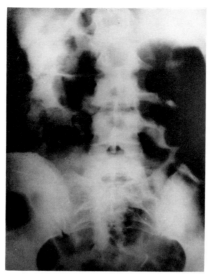

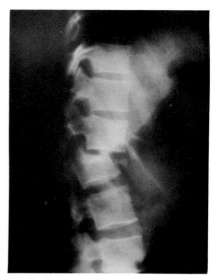

Fig. 13-5. Twenty-six-year-old female with fracture-dislocation of L1-L2. There was progressive paraparesis and gradual incontinence.
A and *B*, Preoperative films. *C* and *D*,
Postoperative results with 80% reduction and
complete neurologic recovery. There was some
residual pain six months postoperatively, which
disappeared after one year.

Fig. 13-5*B*.

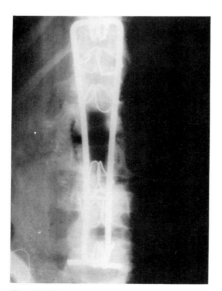

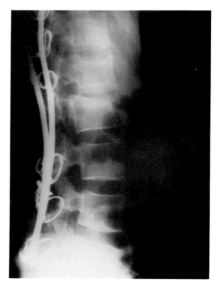

Fig. 13-5*C*.

Fig. 13-5*D*.

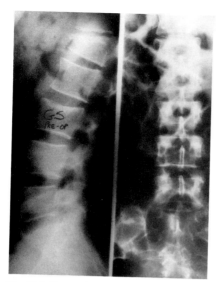

Fig. 13-6. Twenty-four-year-old male with a burst fracture of L1 after falling off a ladder. No neurologic deficit existed. *A,* Preoperative films. *B,* Axial tomogram shows fragment of vertebral body in spinal canal. *C,* Lateral tomogram; arrows show fragment in the canal. *D,* Postoperative axial tomogram. The cancellous bone of the body was resected through the pedicles and the intramedullary fragment tapped into place. *E,* Postoperative lateral tomogram shows patency of neural canal. *F* and *G,* AP and lateral postoperative views.

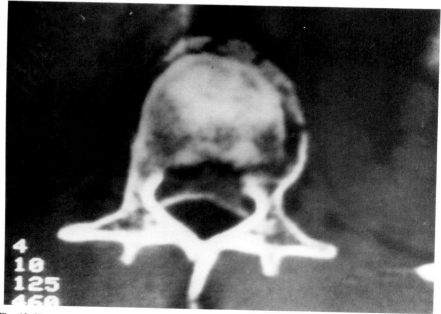

Fig. 13-6*B.*

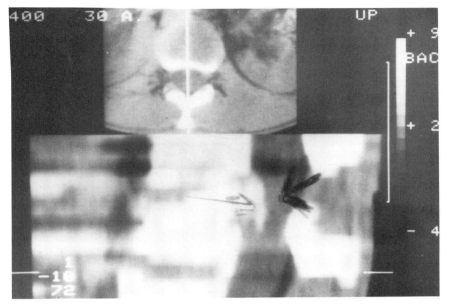

Fig. 13-6*C*.

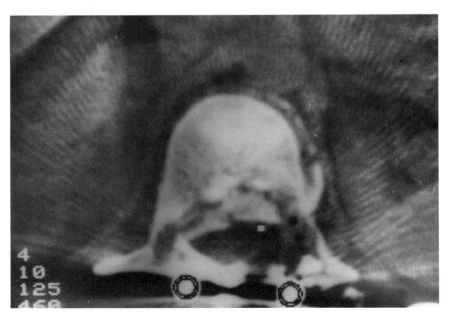

Fig. 13-6*D*.

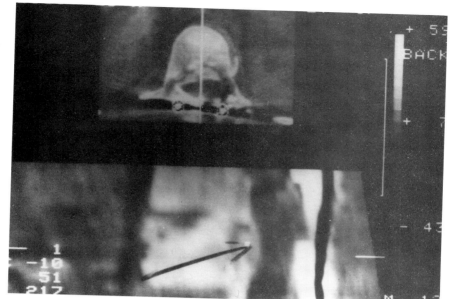

Fig. 13-6E.

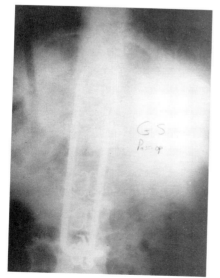

Fig. 13-6F.

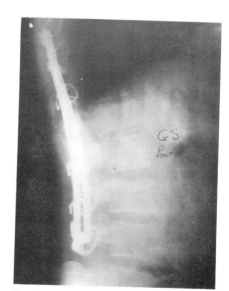

Fig. 13-6G.

Fixation

To avoid using external fixation postoperatively, a rigid internal fixation system consisting of SSI is utilized, as described in the original technique.

The rods are prebent to contour to the normal curves of the spine (kyphosis and lordosis). In the case of paraplegias, hyperlordosis is introduced for better sitting balance and to shift part of the body weight off the ischial tuberosities onto the thighs, thus minimizing pressure sores.

The area of fusion is decided upon in each fracture; in severe compression fractures without laminectomy or neurologic deficit, two segments above and two segments below the fracture are fixed and fused (Fig. 13-5). In fracture-dislocation with laminectomy, corpectomy, or instability, we choose to fix and perform arthrodesis on at least three segments above and below the lesion if there is partial or no neurologic deficit. In paraplegias, the immobilization and arthrodesis are carried down to the sacrum, and hyperlordosis is introduced as stated previously to release pressure from the ischium. This also decreases the energy expenditure during transfers (eg, from bed to wheelchair). In other cases, as in children, we choose not to fuse the area immobilized with SSI because of the growth impairment this will produce.

Results

All our cases without neurologic deficit remained intact postoperatively.

Group I contained ten patients with no neurologic deficit. There were no complications in this group.

Group II consisted of 16 patients with neurologic deficit. Of these, six recovered, two partially and four completely. The remaining ten patients had had complete neurologic lesions since the time of injury and did not recover. All these patients had solidly fused spines by the fourth postoperative month. The complications in this group included one case of a broken rod that, in retrospect, owing to the size of the patient, should have received a 1/4-inch rod; one case of a fracture-dislocation with partial deficit that recovered after complete reduction but lost correction postoperatively (20%), was placed in a Jewett brace, and proceeded to solid fusion; and one last patient with a dislocation of L5 over S1 with fracture of the remaining facets, who had a painful disesthesia in his right leg for three months that resolved spontaneously. No patient had residual pain.

All were seated on the third day postoperatively and were doing transfers and physiotherapy on the tenth postoperative day.

Discussion

This procedure produces rigid internal fixation of the spine, promoting fusion, and also makes alignment of the spine in three dimensions possible by

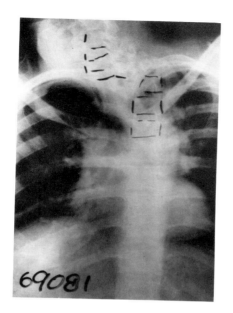

Fig. 13-7. A 32-year-old male who suffered a fracture-dislocation of T12 and T4 falling off a 5-meter scaffold. He is a total paraplegic, with problems on swallowing and in breathing.

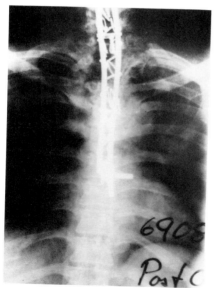

B, After posterior vertebrectomy of T3 with corresponding rib resection, a good alignment is obtained by using the L-rods as lever arms.

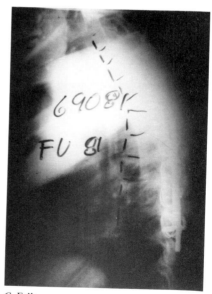

C, Follow-up one year postoperatively, showing good alignment on the lateral x-ray. Patient remains paraplegic but has overcome his respiratory and deglutition deficiencies.

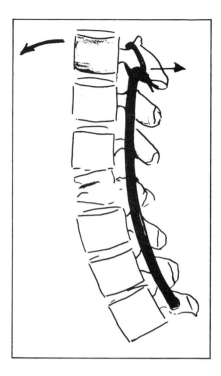

Fig. 13-8. The superior end of the rod is placed in a groove beneath the superior spinous process to avoid posterior migration. Three vertebrae above the lesion are immobilized and three below. Normal lordosis for an L1 fracture is incorporated into the system.

using the rods as lever arms. The fixation is obtained by a three-point fixation: rods and wire on the laminae, and the disk in front as the third fixation point. Using segmental fixation in these patients, we have a method of support that generally does not need external immobilization and promotes arthrodesis.

Editor's Commentary

It is usually hard to maintain reduction of fracture-dislocations with instability (Denis), unless the SSI is done laterally and as far forward as possible, not next to the spinous process. In some of these fractures, not only are shortening procedures and lever arms (SSI rods) needed to reduce the deformity, but also occasionally traction must be applied with an outrigger (Fig. 13-7). In any collapsing spine, a closed-rod system must be used to maintain the length and the correction of the spine.

Fracture-dislocations with a rotational component must be fixed after being reduced with a square or rhomboid bar (if the sacrum is included), which is placed well in front of the facet joints. In my experience, this type of fracture requires both anterior and posterior fusion.

Most SSI systems used to correct kyphosis must be bent underneath bone (eg, spinous process at the ends, since this is the point of maximum workload on the system) (Fig. 13-8). Double wires should be tightened with a "wire hook;" otherwise the tension put on one wire will never be equal to that on the other wire (Fig. 13-8).

In fractures, the concept of fusing only the area of pathologic changes seems very attractive, and in our hands in a limited number of patients has been highly successful. The SSI fixation can then be maintained as long as is necessary to maintain correction and physiologic axial curves. Once the area of pathologic changes undergoes arthrodesis, the fixation can be removed, and flexibility of the unfused spine will resume.

The question regarding the production of arthritis in immobilized joints is not totally answered. There is one thing in favor of SSI: It maintains the facets in a physiologic position, and the muscles around it are normal and are being used continuously during the time of immobilization.

We have had the opportunity to examine facet joints that have been immobilized in this manner more than a year, and they have shown no signs of arthritis. Six patients who have been treated with local fusion, long SSI, and removal of the immobilization one year postoperatively have regained their mobility symptom-free. Although the follow-up and the number of patients in this category are not statistically significant, the idea seems intriguing.

Paraplegic patients must be thought of as totally independent, especially with the advent of the reciprocal swivel walker that has been developed at Oswestry.[6] Anything that will reduce the effort of moving their paralyzed extremities should be done.

Patients who have a history of progressive neurologic posttrauma involvement, even if they seem to be complete paraplegics on admission, should be treated as emergencies. The cord may be tethered or compressed, but if it is aligned and decompressed, some neurologic function may return.

References

1. Luque ER: Personal communication.

2. Rockwood CA, Green DP: Fractures, Vol. 2. Philadelphia, PA, J.B. Lippincott Co., 1975, pp 861-897.

3. Luque ER: The correction of postural curves of the spine. Spine 7(3):270-275, 1982.

4. Luque ER, Cassis N, Ramirez-Wiella G: Segmental Spinal Instrumentation in the treatment of fractures of the thoracolumbar spine. Spine 7(3):312-317, 1982.

5. DeWald RL, Rodts MF, Fister JS: The Management of Burst Fractures of the Thoracic and Lumbar Spine. Exhibit at the American Academy of Orthopedic Surgeons, Anaheim, California, 1983.

6. Farmer IR, Pointer R, Rose CK, Patrich H: The adult swivel walker. Ambulation for paraplegic and tetraplegic patients. Paraplegia 20:248-254, 1982.

Complications in Segmental Spinal Instrumentation

14

Introduction

Segmental spinal instrumentation (SSI) has become firmly established as an effective means of spinal fixation, especially in the management of difficult spinal deformity problems. The complications discussed in this chapter were observed during four years' experience (more than 130 procedures of segmental spinal instrumentation) at our institution. Unlike some centers, however, we have not entirely discarded Harrington instrumentation, which, in combination with spinal fusion, has been used successfully more than 20 years.[1] We still use it for routine idiopathic scoliosis in adolescents and in most cases of uncomplicated scoliosis in adults. Complications of spinal instrumentation in idiopathic curves using the Harrington technique are low.[2] In these curves, both SSI and Harrington instrumentation can be relied on to give adequate correction, to hold that correction, and to allow spinal arthrodesis. The main advantage of the SSI is the ability to offer the patient reduced or no postoperative immobilization. The time during which the patients have been kept in a cast or polypropylene brace after Harrington instrumentation, however, has been greatly liberalized, and at this early stage in the evolution of SSI, we do not believe that the difference in the length of postoperative immobilization is important enough to justify multiple laminotomies and sublaminal wiring, as is required in the SSI technique. Patients view the risk of even trivial neurologic damage as twice as important as wearing a cast.[3]

Segmental spinal instrumentation has expanded and enhanced our ability to deal effectively with difficult spinal problems, including patients with severe degrees of deformity, those with muscle weakness and poor respiratory function, those with osteoporosis due to immobilization or any disorders causing weak bone stock, and those with mental retardation who are unable to comply with postoperative instructions. The incidence of complications in such patients will inevitably be higher than in adolescents with idiopathic scoliosis. Therefore, the complications described here are, in many cases, not directly related to the type of instrumentation. Methods used in the treatment of these patients before the introduction of SSI had a similar higher incidence of complications than in the treatment of idiopathic scoliosis in adolescents.[4]

Complications may be divided into the following headings: (1) component, (2) mechanical, and (3) clinical or physiologic. Many complications, however, have their basis in a combination of two or more of these factors. Neurologic complications remain the greatest concern.

Neurologic Complications

Paraplegia, Complete or Incomplete

This catastrophic complication has devastating effects on both the ambulatory patient and the nonambulatory, wheelchair-bound patient. The former will be severely affected by loss of sensation, and of bowel or bladder control. Management may be made much more difficult because of pressure areas, recurring urinary tract infections, and deformities arising from spasticity.

Incidence

Luque has reported an incidence of 4.6% transient and 0.6% permanent neurologic sequelae after SSI with fusion, and a 2.5% incidence in SSI without fusion.[5] At Children's Hospital in New Orleans, more than 100 SSI procedures were done during the last four years, with four neurologic complications, an incidence of 4%.

There was no spinal injury in a further 35 procedures done in adults during that period. In all cases, the neurologic deficit was initially profound, and the patients have partially recovered. The following common factors were seen in these cases: (1) Kyphosis: two of the four cases involved correction of kyphosis, one of which was a Type I congenital kyphosis in a 19-year-old man who had presented with a partial neurologic deficit. The SSI was preceded by anterior vertebrectomy and fibular strut grafting. (2) Anterior surgery: two of the four patients had undergone an anterior procedure without instrumentation. (3) Three of the four patients suffered from epileptic seizures. In two cases, grand mal seizures occurred in the early postoperative phase.

These factors compare with the high-risk situations for neurologic catastrophe outlined by the Scoliosis Research Society, namely congenital scoliosis, kyphosis, scoliosis with severe deformity, pre-existing neurologic deficit, and neurologic deficit acquired in skeletal traction.[6]

Cord Contusion from Sublaminar Wires

There are a number of possible causes for neurologic complications. Cord or nerve root contusion may occur during wire passage, or from inadvertent pressure on the wires in the interval before they are tightened down to the rod. Wire passage is usually well controlled. The greatest risk of contusion occurs after the wires have been passed. The surgeon or assistant may inadvertently lean on wires, causing them to be pushed against the cord or, in the lumbar region, against the cauda equina. For this reason, crimping of the wire around the lamina immediately after wire passage is extremely important. Various wire-holding devices have also been used to minimize manipulation of the wires after passage. Facetectomy should have been completed before wire passage. Another dangerous time is when the rod is being laid in place and the wires are being tightened around the rod. Every effort must be made to precontour the rod to the curve as accurately as possible. Final adjustments in contouring with the bender in a partially wired-in rod is dangerous. Upward pressure should be applied as the wires are being twisted. Occasionally, as the rod is being wired in, both ends of the wire at one level may be found to be lying lateral to the rod. Great care is needed in manipulating one end of that wire to the medial side of the rod. In many cases, it is safer simply to remove the wire at that level. Similarly, if a wire at one level has been overtightened and breaks, it should be removed, and no further attempts should be made to pass another wire at that level with the rod already lying in place.

The potential for neurologic damage due to wire passage will depend on the relative amount of free space taken up by the wires. The amount of free space, in turn, will depend on the canal diameter and the size of the wires. With the passage of time, the free space in the canal may be lost further because of fibrosis developing around the wires or degenerative changes in the spine. The canal may also possibly narrow because of hypertrophy through a posterior fusion mass.[7] It is difficult to determine how important wire size is in the potential for neurologic disturbance. A recent study of segmental wiring in beagle dogs showed that all six dogs used had a neurologic deficit. The gross specimens had "a magnitude of injury not previously suspected," including indentations of the dura by the wires and severe epidural and subdural hemorrhages.[8] In a study designed to test growth potential of the spine with SSI, the first three beagles in the pilot study became paraplegic as a result of the use of double 16-gauge wires. When smaller wires were used, the animals had no further neurologic compromise.[9] Beagles are dysmorphic, although not as severely so as dachshunds or basset hounds.

One lesson from these studies is that SSI should be used with great caution in humans in conditions such as achondroplasia or other conditions in which there is an acquired or developmental narrow canal.[10] More important, these studies show that if the canal size is marginal, the size of wires assumes some importance. In the standard segmental wiring technique, single 16-gauge wires are used on each side of each level, with doubled 16-gauge wires at the ends. At present, the author is using doubled 18-gauge wires on each side at each level to avoid cut ends of wires and to allow use of the swivel wire tightener, which he prefers. Other centers have used double 20-gauge wires at each level. Although smaller gauge wire is desirable from a neurologic point of view, its use must be weighed against mechanical wire failure. Wire failure with single 18-gauge wires at each level prompted Luque to move to single 16-gauge wires.

The diameter of the wires is not the sole determinant of decreased canal space. Fibrous tissue will develop around the wires, further narrowing the canal, as Gillespie described in his studies in pigs.[11] In addition, he noted grooving of the dura in the sacrificed animal, although the pigs had remained neurologically intact.

Contusion During Wire Removal

Removal may be required either in the acute situation in which the cortical evoked potential has changed, or in the chronic situation, for pain, paresthesia, infection, mechanical failure, or rod protuberance. The two situations differ in that in the late wire removal, the rods will have already formed fibrous tissue tunnels. A unique study of wire removal in cadaver spines undergoing instrumentation with SSI was recently reported.[12] They compared three methods of removing the wires—a vertical pull, pulling as horizontally as possible, and winding the wires up. They showed instances of compression of the dura in 30% of the wire removals. It was found in all methods of wire removal, and particularly if the wire was wound up. In some cases, the wire whiplashed to the point of coming in contact with the posterior longitudinal ligament.

The following procedures are advised for minimizing the possibility of neurologic damage during removal. First, cut the end of the wire that is to be pulled through as close to the bone as possible, avoiding a long tail, which could flip forward. Second, the wires usually lie in an elliptical fashion beneath the lamina. They should be pulled out as much as possible along the curve of that ellipse, probably midway between a vertical and a horizontal position. Third, use a slow, steady movement.

Neurologic Damage Due to Cord Stretch or Distraction

Segmental spinal instrumentation has often been said to have a greater corrective force in severe curves than the Harrington distraction method. From a biomechanical point of view, this theory may not be correct, but the SSI method is certainly able to maintain large corrective forces that may be applied to the spine. Indeed, the greater the correction that is accomplished, the smaller the residual curve and the lower the stress at each fixation point.[13] There is less opportunity to "feel" the amount of force being imparted, compared with Harrington distraction rods. Overcorrection may lead to cord stretch and neurologic damage. Care must be taken if a portion of the curve being corrected is rigid. In these cases, correction may be gained maximally at the compensatory curves above and below the rigid segment, drawing the cord firmly in to the apex. Such rigidity is seen, in particular, in kyphosis and was possibly the cause of one case of transient paraplegia in our series. For cord stretch to be avoided whenever possible, the corrective procedure should lead to a shortening in the length of the spine.[5] In rigid segments, this shortening may be possible only by both anterior and posterior surgery.

Because of the great security of fixation with SSI, one is tempted to try to stabilize with a single posterior surgical procedure, ignoring the time-honored principles of spine surgery that require gaining mobility in rigid segments of the curve by anterior release with or without instrumentation. The amount of correction to aim for is difficult to decide at the time of the surgery. For this reason, decisions should be made based on assessment of the x-ray views before surgery. The standard guidelines are for correction to 10 degrees greater than that achieved with the best forced bend. This can be done by making templates from the x-ray film preoperatively. In complex curves, interpretation of bending films may be difficult due to severe rotation. In these cases, we make our bending films with the patient in traction on the Risser table to assure that the shoulders and pelvis are in the same plane. No guidelines have yet been set for the ideal amount of correction of kyphosis. In our experience, kyphosis has been the more troublesome curve from the point of view of neurologic injury. Similar guidelines to those given for scoliosis should apply.

Neurologic Damage Due to Vascular Causes

Two of the four patients in our series in whom neurologic compromise developed had prior anterior release and bone grafting followed by two weeks in halo gravity traction before the posterior SSI procedure. Although care was taken to tie off the segmental vessels as anteriorly as possible to preserve the vascular arcade around the foramen, the possibility remains that disturbance of the vasculature anteriorly

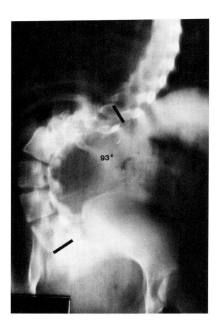

Fig. 14-1A. This patient is a 22-year-old female, fully ambulatory, with mental retardation of unknown origin. She had a rapidly progressive complex spinal curvature leading to increasing decompensation and pelvic obliquity. The scoliosis measured 98 degrees from T11 to L5 (A). Over the same segment there was a kyphosis of 63 degrees, with a compensatory lordosis in the thoracic spine (B). Initial surgery consisted of anterior discectomy and bone grafting from T11-12 through L3-4. This was followed by three weeks of halo gravity traction. The second stage consisted of SSI from T3-sacrum. There was approximately 50% correction in both the scoliosis and the kyphosis (C and D) Corticosensory evoked potentials remained unchanged throughout the procedure. Postoperatively the patient was neurologically intact to careful examination. However, on the sixth day she was noted to be paraplegic with only some residual deep sensation in the right leg. Corticosensory evoked potentials were absent in the left leg and present in the right leg, but with a greatly decreased amplitude and delayed latency.

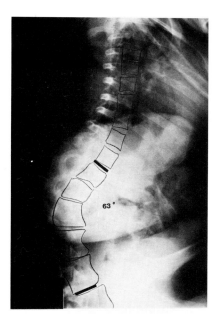

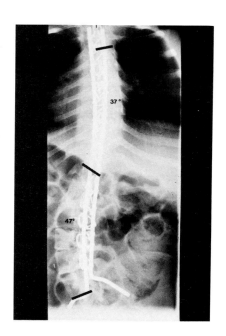

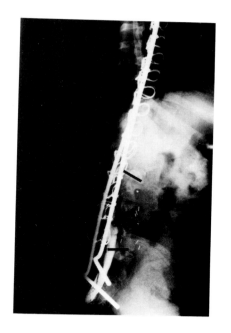

may preset the cord to the potential for neurologic damage at the second procedure. The fact that the segmental vascular supply to the cord is uneven, with some levels contributing very little and other levels having major feeders, has led some authors to suggest preoperative vertebral angiography to identify the major spinal cord feeders. When there is a marginal vascular supply, profound hypotensive episodes in the immediate postoperative period may have serious detrimental effect. Hypotensive episodes may occur during grand mal seizures. The secure fixation of SSI allows early wheelchair sitting postoperatively in neuromuscular scoliosis cases, which is of great benefit in preventing pulmonary complications and preventing accelerated muscle weakness in muscular dystrophy. In some patients with neurologic disorders, however, normal vascular reflexes are often decreased or absent. Patients may be unable to voice feelings of dizziness or faintness when they are sat up, and profound hypotension may occur. Such episodes may possibly initiate or worsen neurologic function in a patient with marginal cord blood supply.

Neurologic Deficits and Spinal Cord Monitoring

We have been routinely using cortical somatosensory-evoked monitoring techniques. A number of false-positive recordings have been made, but no false-negative recordings. Of great concern, however, is that in all four cases of neurologic injury, the paraplegia was of delayed onset. Findings on neurologic examination were normal in the immediate postoperative phase, but paraplegia developed in an interval between 48 hours and five days. Spinal cord monitoring was used on three of these patients. Prolonged latency was seen in only one.

Delayed onset of paraplegia has previously been reported with Harrington instrumentation.[14] Such delayed onset, in one case, highlighted the danger of relying too heavily on spinal cord monitoring. In that case, the rods were wired in slowly, with constant reference to the monitor. Correction to a greater degree than that outlined by the principles given previously was selected, and normal intraoperative spinal cord monitor trace and normal findings on postoperative neurologic examination gave the surgeon a false confidence. Based on these experiences, the spinal cord monitor should not be used as the arbiter of the degree of curve correction selected (Fig. 14-1).

Other Disturbance to the Dural Sac and Neural Elements

Dural tear. With careful technique in making the laminotomy, dural tears are not common. The area most likely to tear is the S1-S2 interspace when rods are being wired to the pelvis. The dura here is thin, and epidural fat is minimal. This complication should be handled in a manner similar to a dural tear with any other spinal procedures.[15] The laminotomy must be widened and the tear carefully closed with a fine dural stitch. A small fascial graft may sometimes be necessary. Ignoring a cerebrospinal fluid leak may lead to cerebrospinal fluid fistula, with its attendant risk of meningitis, or the formation of a pseudomeningocele with entrapment of the nerve roots.

Epidural bleeding. Epidural bleeding can often be avoided if the laminotomies are carefully made. If the epidural veins are distended, bleeding will be difficult to avoid. For this reason, the patient must be checked before surgery to ensure that the abdomen is free from pressure. Epidural bleeding is more common in cases of severe hypokyphosis, in which the cord tends to run in the back of the spinal canal with very little epidural fat. A small piece of gelfoam soaked in thrombin covered by cottonoid is usually sufficient to control most epidural bleeding. Both the cottonoid and the gelfoam should, however, be removed. The laminotomies should prevent epidural hematoma formation; however, if the large pieces of gelfoam are placed at each level and kept in place, a seal may develop that may allow a significant epidural hematoma to form.

Nerve root foraminal impingement. A few patients complain postoperatively of neuralgia, numbness, or sciatica, which appears to be in a fairly well demarcated nerve root distribution. In the author's experience, adults are more likely to be affected. In most cases, the impingement settles spontaneously and is no longer a problem. In one adult patient, persistent neuralgia in a T12 distribution abated only when the rods were removed one year after their insertion. The patient fortunately had a solid fusion at that stage. In correction of kyphosis, hyperesthesia of the anterior chest or abdominal wall may be seen but is usually transient. It is

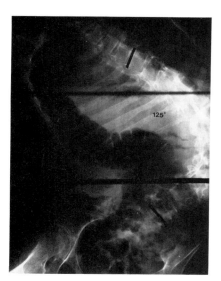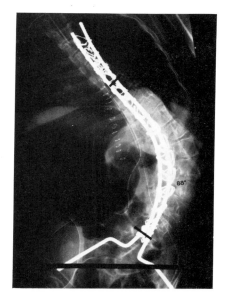

Fig. 14-2*A & B* A 22 year old nonambulatory patient with mental retardation and progressive scoliosis. There was increasing pelvic obliquity causing loss of seating balance. The preoperative curve measured 125 degrees (I). Preoperative bending films appeared to show correction to 65 degrees (II). However, at surgery, the curve was found to be rigid with virtual ankylosis of the concave facets. SSI was carried out with little correction of the primary curve. The Biophase rods were selected. The final correction was 88 degrees (III). Despite disappointing correction, stabilization has been sufficient to allow the patient to sit in an adapted wheelchair.

On reflection, the pre-op bending film was probably misleading due to rotation that occurred with the lateral bending. Bending rods to conform to this degree of curvature causes dangerous loading, and may result in rod breakage.

accompanied by anterior rib pain and appears to be related to forcible stretching out of the tissues between the ribs, rather than nerve root impingement.[16]

Complications Due to Component Failures

Rod Breakage

As with Harrington instrumentation, rod breakage usually indicates an underlying pseudarthrosis. The fatigue strength of the rod is determined by its diameter and the composition of the alloy. Rods are available in stainless steel in diameters of $\frac{3}{16}''$

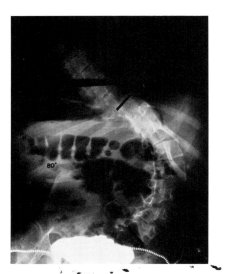 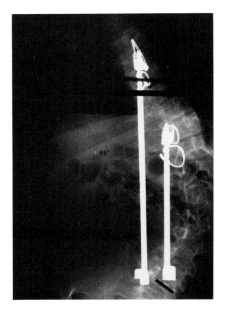

Fig. 14-2*C & D* A 16 year old male with spinal muscular atrophy, presented with progressive scoliosis and pelvic obliquity. His preoperative curve was 80 degrees. Pulmonary function studies were poor, with the forced vital capacity being 23% of the predicted value. For this reason, combined anterior and posterior procedures were thought to be contraindicated. Two weeks of halo gravity traction failed to reduce the curvature, but pulmonary function tests increased to around 40% of predicted values. The patient underwent a posterior procedure with intended SSI fixation. At surgery the curvature was found to be rigid with very little correctability. Rather than bend Luque rods excessively to conform to the large curvature, doubled Harrington rods were inserted on the concavity, with segmental wiring to help anchor the hooks. Postoperatively the patient required two weeks before being able to be weaned off ventilatory support, but since has gone on the solid fusion without further progression.

and ¼″, and also in cobalt-nickel alloy in ³⁄₁₆″. Rods ³⁄₁₆″ in diameter have been recommended for use in myelodysplasia and idiopathic and neuromuscular scoliosis. The quarter-inch rods have been recommended in fracture cases, revisions, and kyphosis.

Rod breakage has not been a major problem with SSI. Most cases have occurred when excessive bends have been incorporated into the rods to allow them to conform to large curvatures. This fact again outlines the importance of correcting curvatures by release procedures, either anteriorly, posteriorly, or both, before definitive posterior instrumentation. During the early stages of SSI use, fear of rod breakage led to an excessive reliance on the quarter-inch rods. The two sizes of rods, however, have vastly different working properties. Quarter-inch rods are extremely inflexible and must be contoured precisely to the spine. Such contouring is especially difficult if a number of bends must be made in the rods, as in the Galveston pelvic fixation. The lack of flexibility also appears to put added stress on the wires, leading to increased wire breakage. For this reason, $\frac{3}{16}''$ rods are now used in all situations except where severe loading may be anticipated, as in spinal fractures in adults and in kyphosis in adults. Wherever possible, the surgeon should avoid contouring the rod to match a curve greater than 60 to 70 degrees, particularly over a short segment. Although the posterior elements will have less of a curvature than the vertebral bodies, segmental spinal instrumentation is much less effective in this situation. Some patients with a severe established deformity have a pulmonary status that makes anterior releasing procedures unfeasible. In these cases, we have used halo gravity traction followed by posterior instrumentation alone, to avoid progression. In these situations, Harrington distraction rods are biomechanically more advantageous in gaining correction but have the need for external mobilization and carry the risk of loss of fixation at the hook sites. Segmental spinal fixation has the disadvantages of poor biomechanical correctibility and weakening of the rods due to incorporation to conform to a large curve. If segmental spinal instrumentation is selected, the cobalt-nickel alloy should be used (Fig. 14-2).

Rod Migration or Rotation

Vertical slipping of rods leads to loss of the decussation between the rods at the ends. This decussation, along with the horizontal wires between the rods at three levels, firmly binds the concave and convex rods together and closes the "loop." As the spine deformity is being corrected, some increase in length should be anticipated and provided for by allowing about an inch of overlap above and below in the length to both rods. The short horizontal limb should lie deep to the long limb of the opposite rod. It should lie in a groove in the spinous process or through a hole in the spinous process; it should not lie simply in the interlaminar area. The lower doubled-end wires are tightened to hold the rods in position. Rods are less likely to migrate or slip with instrumentation over long spine segments and when sagittal curves are incorporated into the rods. The complications are more common in short segments. Instrumentation over a short segment does little to control rotation. For this reason, in short segments, bilateral C-rods wired together in a closed-box configuration are preferable. Ready-made box configuration rods are now being manufactured in various lengths.

    Small amounts of rod migration rarely cause serious problems (Fig. 14-3). When the migration occurs from the thoracic into the lumbar area, however, the rod end often becomes palpable beneath the skin in the region of the lumbar lordosis, and a painful bursa may form over the end. This problem is difficult to treat. Cutting off the horizontal end leaves the rod straight, and it will surely slip further. These cases may be salvaged by using the recently developed locking device, a

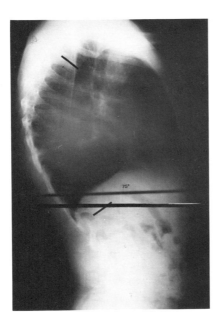

Fig. 14-3A. This is an eighteen year old male with persistent pain and deformity from Scheuermann's kyphosis. The kyphosis measured 75 degrees, correcting to 58 degrees on forced extension. There was vertebral wedging of 10 degrees over four levels. He underwent staged procedures, the first being anterior discectomy and bone grafting, followed by halo gravity traction for two weeks. The second stage was posterior SSI from T2–L2, using 1/4″ rods. Postoperative correction was to 53 degrees (B). It should be noted that the lower end of the rods are incorrectly seated in the interlaminal area and are well below the double end wires (B and C). At six months slippage was noted. This progressed, and at one year, the rod was prominent in the lumbar area, with a symptomatic bursa associated with it. The lower end wire had broken (D and E).

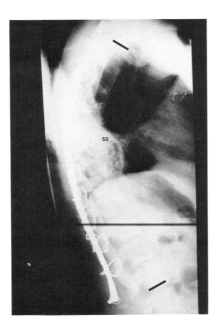

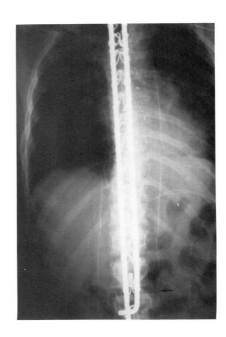

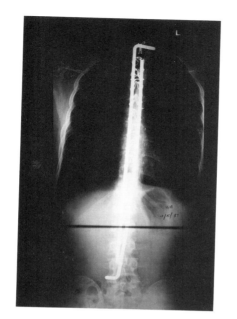
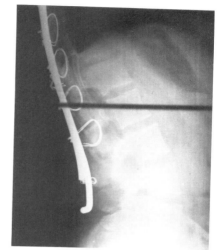

collar that can be secured to the rod and the sublaminal wire at the end of the L-rod, preventing migration.[17]

Wire Breakage

The cause of wire breakage, which is not uncommon with SSI, may often rest with improper technique rather than with the property of the wires. At the completion of the wire procedure, the rod should rest on the laminae firmly against the base of the spinous process. The wire should not be twisted to approximate a rod to a lamina, nor should attempts be made to pull the spine to the rod. The wires should be tightened to secure the position of the rod at the base of the lamina. For this reason, wire breakage seems more common with the use of 1/4-inch rods, which, because of their stiffness, are much harder to get to conform to the spine.

Experience shows that the wires usually break at the ends of instrumentation, and for this reason, double wires should be used on both sides above and below. Because of the special forces on the end wires, the cut ends tend to rotate into the vertical position and become prominent under the skin. For this reason, the ends should be left a little longer than the interculary wires. After the ends are bent over, a small horizontal wire is used to secure them. The wire twists should be evenly applied, rather than a wire wrap. Wire achieves its full strength at three twists, with a pitch of three twists to a centimeter.[18]

Laminar Erosion

Fatigue testing of SSI in cadaver spines has shown a significant degree of laminar erosion. This change is difficult to see on x-ray film. The clinical significance of laminar erosion is uncertain, and one would expect it to be much less prominent in spines that have undergone solid fusion.

Kyphosis Occurring at the Top of the Segment Undergoing Instrumentation

This phenomenon has been seen both in neuromuscular curves and in spines fused for Scheuermann's kyphosis. Several mechanisms may cause this problem. First, and most commonly, the segment undergoing instrumentation has been stopped too short, especially in the collapsing kyphoscoliosis seen in neuromuscular conditions. In these cases, even if the upper end point of the kyphosis appears to be the midthoracic level, extension of the rods to T2 or T3 is advocated. Above the instrumentation is a stress riser, the junction of a mobile and an immobile segment. Concentration of stresses here may lead to some weakening of the ligamentous tissues and consequently some fall-off. This situation may be exacerbated by muscular weakening due to paraspinous muscle stripping and unnecessary removal of ligaments above the level undergoing instrumentation. The progression of fall-off above the level undergoing instrumentation appears to be maximum at three to six months after surgery. The top wires might break or slide off the rods, and the rods themselves may become prominent under the skin. In patients who have fusions of adequate length and who have head control, however, we have found progression of the kyphosis spontaneously arrests after about a year, and revision is usually not required (Fig. 14-4). Similarly, at a lower end of the rods, pelvic obliquity may occasionally progress sharply in neuropathic curves in which fusion stops short of the sacrum. For this reason, the spines of all nonambulatory patients with neuromuscular problems should be fused to the sacrum.

Corrosion at the Rod-Wire Interface

In the early weeks after SSI, before the spinal fusion has taken hold, minute motion will occur at each segment between the rod and the wire. With this motion, metal will rub against metal, producing microfragments. This process greatly increases the surface area between the metal and the body's tissues. This situation, which is similar to that seen after the McKee-Farrara total hip replacements, may possibly in susceptible persons lead to problems with metal sensitivity, particularly in the use of the cobalt-nickel alloy.[19,20] Anecdotal reports have been made of severe staining seen around the rod-wire interface after SSI. On a number of revisions, however, the author has found staining to be rarely present and, when seen, to be slight.

Pseudarthrosis

Early in its development, concern over whether the rate of solid fusion would be much lower with SSI than with the Harrington technique was considerable for several reasons. The space taken up by the fixation was increased. Decortication of the laminae was avoided, for fear of weakening the segmental wire attachments. It was desirable to avoid excising the entire spinous process, to prevent rod migration. The standard Moe facet fusion was avoided because of the possibility that increased bleeding would obscure visualization of wire passage. Finally, the technique has been used in many patients with poor bone stock and wafer-thin iliac crests.

In practice, most surgeons have been gratified by the high rate of fusion seen with the technique. The fusion techniques differ with different authors. The Galveston technique is to avoid laminar decortication or facet excision and to use large volumes of bone graft along the costotransverse processes in the thoracic spine and lateral to the facet joints as far as the transverse processes in the lumbar spine. Support for this approach comes from revisions, in which the bulk of the fusion mass is invariably found lateral to the rods. The large callus response seen with SSI may be related to the fact that the fixation is secure, but not rigid. In this way, it may act like semi-rigid plates in long bone fractures. If this theory is correct, it argues against a trend toward thicker or more rigid rods.

Sacroiliac Joint Pain

This complication has been seen in a number of patients whose spines have been fused to the pelvis. Currently practiced forms of pelvic fixation cross the sacroiliac joint but do not formally arthrodese them (Fig. 14-5). In my experience, sacroiliac joint pain has been seen mainly in nonambulatory patients who have high-demand sitting, for example, patients with spinal muscular atrophy who hold down jobs sitting at a desk for long periods. Sacroiliac joint pain has also been reported in adult patients who have had segmental spinal instrumentation and fusion to the sacrum for lumbar degenerative disease.[21] Diagnosis can be made by careful questioning of the patient. A definite pattern of sacroiliac pain will be elicited, separate from the other aches and pains that these patients get from time to time. It has the characteristic location, is made worse by cold weather and activity, and is eased by rest and anti-inflammatory medication. The pain can be reproduced by the Fabere or Gaenslen's tests. The symptoms are most severe in the period six months to one year after surgery and tend to abate after that. They have not reached the stage at which revision has been required. Efforts have been made to develop a form of fixation to the sacrum that does not require instrumentation crossing the sacroiliac joint. This approach, however, may lead to unprotected stresses being localized at the sacroiliac joint. In many cases, where rods cross the sacroiliac joint, the joints appear to undergo attrition or ankylosis.

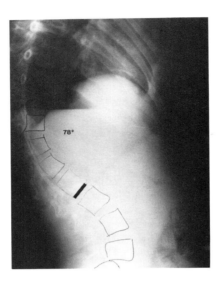
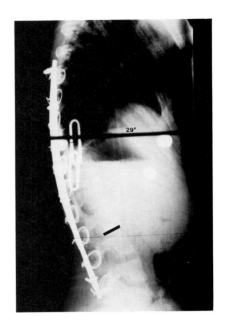

Fig. 14-4A. A fifteen year old female with Noonan's syndrome was noted to have a progressive kyphosis. Preoperatively this measured 79 degrees from T9-L2. She underwent a simultaneous anterior and posterior fusion. SSI was carried out posteriorly from T7-L5, and disc removal and interbody fusion carried out anteriorly from T11-L2. *B.* Postoperative curvature was 29 degrees. *C.* Twenty months postoperatively the anterior fusion was solid, and the correction maintained, but fall-off had occurred through the upper part of the instrumented segment with wire breakage. The case was revised by removing the rods only, and replacing them with longer 1/4″ rods, placed in the caudal direction along the existing fiberosseous tunnels. Four levels were added to the top. CFTRID. An eighteen year old female with mental retardation and progressive scoliosis. Her preoperative scoliosis measured 84 degrees. There was not significant kyphosis. *E. This shows the lateral x-ray at the upper part of the rod following spine fusion from T2-sacrum. F.* Lateral x-ray 12 months later showing fall-off occurring above the instrumented segment, with loss of the top wire fixation. However, the patient had good head control and no further progression of kyphosis occurred. The rods did not become prominent under the skin and an excellent clinical result has been maintained.

Loss of Pelvic Fixation

The Galveston fixation to the pelvis appears to be the most secure. We have had one case of loss of fixation. This case involved an immature, nonambulatory child with severe mental retardation and severe kyphoscoliosis. Excellent correction was gained, and about one month postoperatively the child's normal physical therapy regimen, which involved vigorously treating the extension contractures in his hips with forceful hip flexion, was reapplied. The physical therapy caused the whole pelvis to rotate forward, pulling the rods from the pelvic fixation and leaving them prominent under the skin posteriorly (Fig. 14-6).

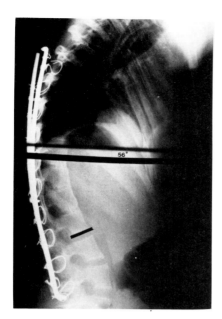
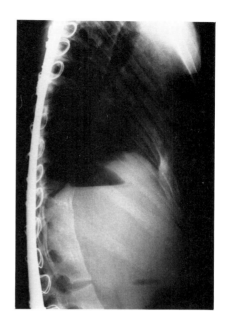

Pelvic Fixation, a Detriment to Ambulation?

This question arose after a series of patients having neuromuscular scolioses, mainly polio patients, were reported to have decreased ability to walk after SSI with pelvic fixation.[22] This problem fortunately is not common. Most neuropathic curves progress to the stage of requiring surgery when the patient's condition deteriorates to the point at which most of his time is spent in a wheelchair. This situation is particularly true in muscular dystrophy and to a lesser extent in cerebral palsy. Further observation and research are required before this question can be answered.

Pelvic Obliquity and Cephalopelvic Decompensation

Less than ideal correction of pelvic obliquity and decompensation have been reported with SSI. Lack of distraction of the corrective force in the system has been cited as the most likely explanation.[23] For this reason, we originally used a Harrington outrigger on the concavity of the curve to try to get better correction of the pelvic obliquity. We have since discarded this technique. In neuromuscular scoliosis, in which there is often no lumbar compensatory curve, correction of pelvic obliquity is a function of the correction of the lumbosacral scoliosis. Therefore, approximately 50% correction can be anticipated with the posterior

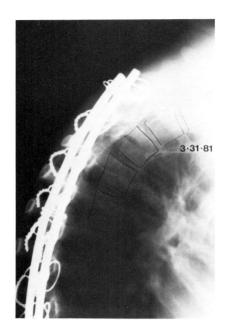

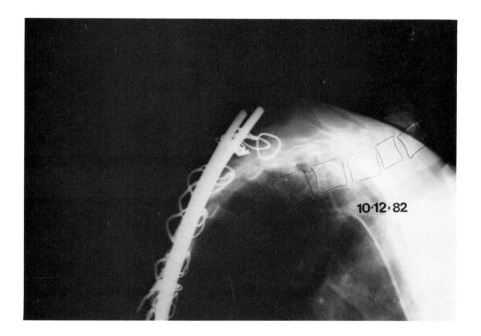

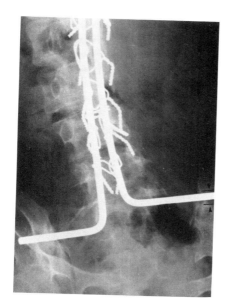

Fig. 14-5. Pelvic fixation used prior to adopting the Galveston method. The rod ends were inserted in holes in the posterior ileum. No wires were used to secure the rods or laminae at the proximal sacrum. Note the windshield wiper effect seen on either side of the right rod. This is also seen commonly around the rod ends with the Galveston fixation.

procedure alone, which is often sufficient for low-demand sitters. In the high-demand sitters, for whom equal pressure on the ischial tuberosities is essential, we use anterior instrumentation with Zielke apparatus followed by posterior SSI. In our hands, this procedure has given the best results (Fig. 14-7).

Medical Complications

Gastrointestinal

Gastroesophageal reflux is common in cerebral palsy and other neuropathic conditions. It may be worsened by spinal surgery. We now do a barium study before SSI in all patients with cerebral palsy. Patients with significant reflux are referred to general surgery, and if necessary fundoplication is done first. Other gastrointestinal problems encountered after SSI include gastric atony and pancreatitis. Interestingly, all cases of superior mesenteric artery syndrome encountered at our institution have been associated with idiopathic curves and Harrington instrumentation.

Infection

The author has seen three cases of infection with SSI. Two became apparent two weeks after the surgery, and a third was seen at one year after the surgery. In the two

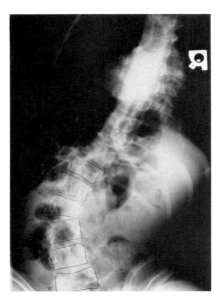 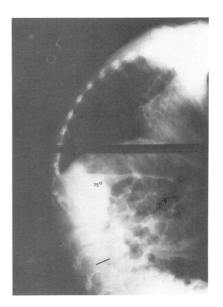

Fig. 14-6. A twelve year old child with mental retardation and recent onset of collapsing kyphosis measuring 75 degrees, with scoliosis measuring 46 degrees and early pelvic obliquity (*A* and *B*). SSI was carried out from T3-sacrum with correction of the scoliosis and a restoration of the sagittal plane curvatures (*C* and *D*). The iliac fixation was compromised by soft bone with a thin inner table to the ileum. The length of the rod into the ileum could have been longer for optimal fixation. The lamina of the first sacral segment was not strong enough to allow fixation to the rod. Six months postop, the pelvis was noted to have tilted forward, with the rods pulling away and becoming prominent under the skin (*E*). This required partial rod removal. One year postop, the patient developed deep infection around the rods, requiring total rod removal. However, a solid fusion was found lateral to the rods from T3-sacrum.

early infections, a hematoma was believed to be the cause. When pelvic obliquity was corrected and lumbar lordosis restored, the skin became stretched over the area between the rib cage and iliac crest, on the concavity. This dead space filled in with blood, and the area became infected. The author now carefully stitches this area down to obliterate the dead space and assure the drain's exit from this area. In the two early postoperative cases, the rods were left in. In one case, debridement and suction perfusion tubes were not helpful. After further debridement and healing by secondary intention, the infection has remained quiescent, and the spine has gone on to solid fusion. In the case of infection presenting at one year, the rods were removed, and a solid spine fusion was found from T3 to the sacrum. All infected patients were incontinent. Special care in the postoperative stage needs to be taken to protect the lower wound from coming in contact with wet diapers. It is now

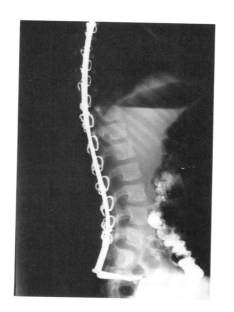

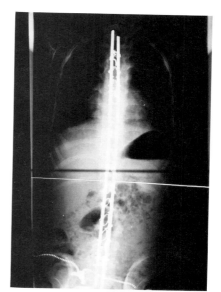

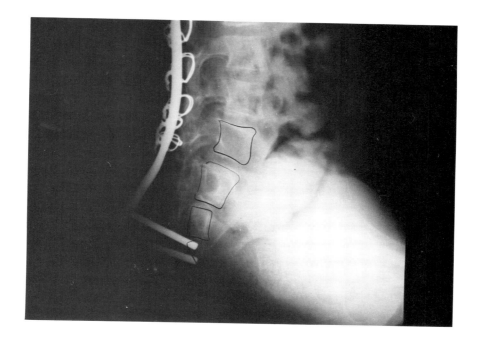

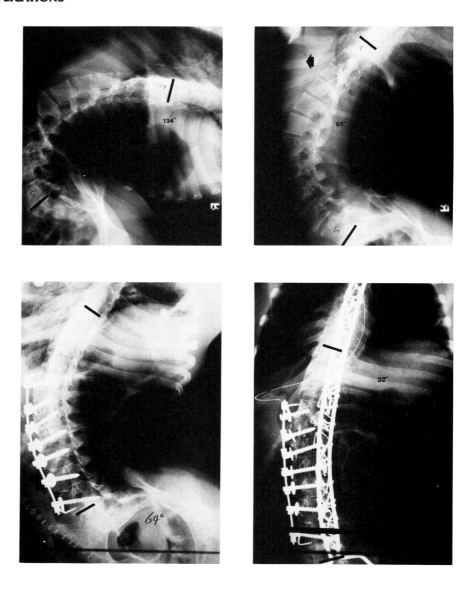

Fig. 14-7. A 20 year old female with spastic quadriplegia and mental retardation, and a severe progressive scoliosis measuring 134 degrees (*A*). Forced bend allowed correction to only 95 degrees (*B*). Due to the magnitude of the curve and severe pelvic obliquity, the patient was unable to be seated in any adaptive wheelchair and for the previous two years, was forced to lie supine on a beanbag. Anterior surgery with discectomy and bone grafting and Zielke fixation reduced the curvature to 64 degrees (*C*). Two weeks later, SSI was performed with final correction to 32 degrees (*D*). The pelvis was nearly level. The patient now tolerates wheelchair sitting with noticeable improvement in appetite, respiratory function and socialization.

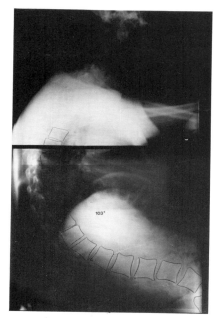 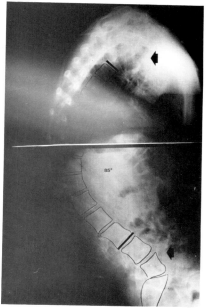

Fig. 14-8. An 18 year old nonambulatory patient with spastic quadriplegia who presented with 103 degree kyphosis (1) correcting to 85 degrees on forced extension (*A*). He underwent staged anterior release and bone grafting, followed by two weeks of halo gravity traction. A second stage SSI was carried out from T3 to the sacrum with final correction of his kyphosis to 51 degrees (*B*). Reversal of his forward pelvis tilt unmasked an extension contracture of his hips, with flexion being allowed to only 60 degrees. This caused difficulty and pain on resumption of wheelchair sitting. Gentle physiotherapy manipulation over the next two months gradually increased his flexion to 90 degrees, allowing comfortable sitting without compromise of pelvic fixation.

policy to do urinalysis and culture before admission for all neuropathic patients with curves and incontinence.

Preexisting Contractures

One of the great advantages of SSI is its ability to correct sagittal plane curvatures, especially in neuromuscular conditions. This may bring to light adaptive changes at either end of the spine, particularly in the neck and hips. The collapsing kyphosis and scoliosis seen in Duchenne muscular dystrophy is commonly accompanied by an extensive contracture of the neck. Correction of kyphosis to the normal degree may lead to inability of the child to have horizontal gaze unless the

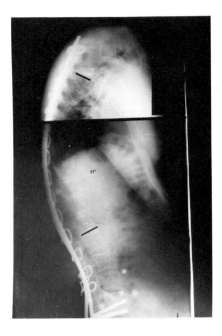

child leans forward in the wheelchair. Established kyphosis, especially in cerebral palsy, often extends down to a forwardly tilted pelvis. Reestablishing the lumbar lordosis and tilting the pelvis back into a more normal position will in many cases unmask an extension contracture at the hips. Inability to flex the hips to 90 degrees causes difficulty in sitting (Fig. 14-8).

Using forceful manipulations in reestablishing 90 degrees of flexion at the hips may jeopardize the pelvic fixation. We have found that gentle postoperative manipulation sufficiently improves the contractures, and operative release of the extensors has not been necessary.

Summary

As the technique of SSI has evolved and has been applied to various spinal problems, complications have arisen. Some complications can be directly related to the instrumentation; others have their basis more in problems inherent in the

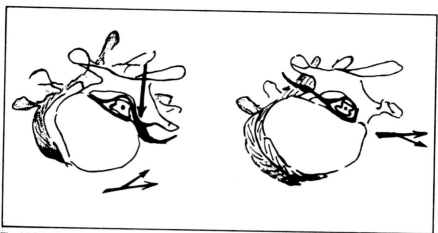

Fig. 14-9A. Elongation of the vertebral column represents an "elongation." The soft tissues, including the blood vessels, are in the concavity of the deformity, and in the case of the aorta and vena cava, are fixed there by the segmental vascular bundles.

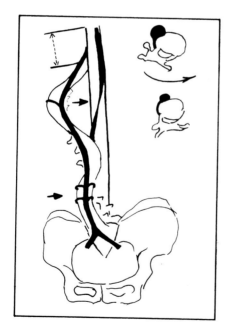

B, Lengthening (by correcting) spinal deformity puts an even larger stretch on the large vessels, forcing a diminution of the lumen. This is true in AP correction, sagittal correction, or axial correction.

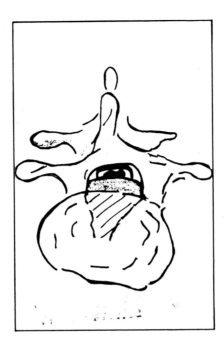

Fig. 14-10A. Obstruction within the neural canal increases the chances of vascular or neurologic injury while trying to correct spinal deformity.

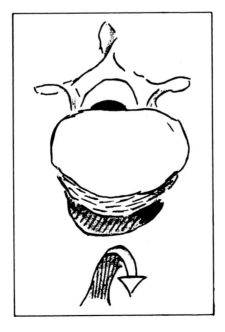

B, A tethered cord in acute kyphosis is already in a borderline situation, and any elongation may produce irreversible damage.

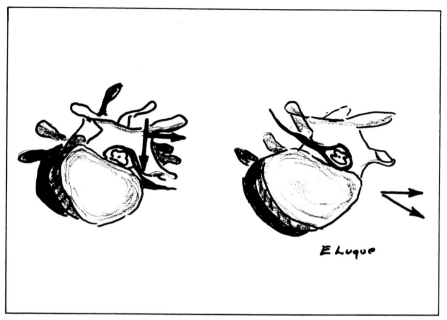

Fig. 14-11. In deformities with a rotational component, entrapment of the concave root or stretching of the convex root is easy to produce, especially with large corrections and with transverse traction. It must be remembered that as spinal pathology is segmental, so are the adaptations of the neural elements.

spine, for which the instrumentation is being used. Because SSI remains a developing field, careful observation and documentation continue to be required.

Editor's Commentary

As SSI has become a common tool to correct and fix spinal deformity, more than the usual number of complications have appeared. Many have occurred in cases that had no effective treatment before SSI.[24,28,29] As a result of this, the length of instrumentation and other technical aspects have been tailored to different problems by trial and error, since no past medical knowledge existed. Many times, errors result from plain surgical incompetence.[25,29] SSI is an exacting technique, not designed for the occasional spine surgeon. The surgical team's familiarity with all the options that the technique offers is necessary to make difficult decisions.

The most feared complication is no doubt neurologic, in the form of partial or complete loss of neural function.[24,25] This can be caused by partial or complete

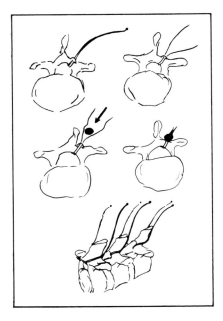

Fig. 14-12. Neurologic damage due to wire impingement on the nerve cord can be avoided by using double closed-looped wire that comes in several lengths for the convenience of the surgeon. It is ideal to use as double wires, tightened with a hook.

It can also be used: 1. by passing the looped end under the lamina. 2. by threading the beaded end through the loop, lassoing the entire lamina. This prevents accidental trauma to the cord and broken surgical gloves during the surgical procedure. 3. by threading the rod in between the long looped wires and snug against the lamina. As the wire is twisted over the rod, the entire system will self-lock.

vascular accident accompanying hypotensive anesthesia or by an episode of hypotension during or immediately after the anesthesia. It can also occur as a direct result of stretching the neural cord while obtaining correction of the deformity; after all, any correction represents a certain amount of lengthening.[24]

Also, before lengthening, we must consider the vascular supply to the neural cord (Fig. 14-9). As the spine is straightened, the vertebral arteries suffer from elongation and decreased cross-sectional lumen size. If in addition segmental derotation is added, the insult can be critical. Sometimes this risk may be increased by doing anterior procedures that require ligation of the segmental vessels over a large area of the spine prior to SSI. There is also a high incidence of anomalous blood supply to the neural cord.

In the correction of kyphosis, these considerations apply, especially with an ischemic tethered cord or anterior bony protrusion into the neural canal (Fig. 14-10A and B).[26] It must also be remembered that due to the nature of the deformity, entrapment of concave roots or stretching of convex roots is easy to provoke (Fig. 14-11). In transposition of the spine, mediastinal axial change can lead to arrhythmias, and too much correction can lead to respiratory deficiencies due to overstretching of the abdominal wall and respiratory muscles.[26] It is well known that a faulty technique that leaves a flat thoracolumbar spine will lead to progressive loss of vital capacity.[26]

Immunologic and hormonal reactions to the surgical trauma and blood replacement have also been recorded as complications. Leaving a patient out of three-dimensional balance, not correcting a thoracolumbar kyphosis, or flattening the lumbar spine is a mistake and consequently results in complications.[27] Using the wrong size rod or wire, inadequate length of fixation, or overworking either rods or wires leads to mechanical failures.[28] Not using looped wires provokes direct contusion or even epidural bleeding around the neural cord (Fig. 14-12).[24] Application of L, C, rectangular, or rhomboidal bars is a surgical judgment but is essential in avoiding pitfalls.[26]

The length of fixation should be determined by the type of deformity— structural, collapsing, degenerative compound scoliotic, or axial.[28] The age of the patient, if still within the growing years or skeletally immature, is also a consideration. Undoubtedly, the most common mistake is overcorrection.[28]

References

1. Harrington PR: Treatment of scoliosis. Correction and internal fixation by spine instrumentation. J Bone Jt Surg 44A:591-610, 1962.

2. Morbidity reports of Scoliosis Research Society.

3. Bunch WH, Chapman RG: Patient preferences in scoliosis surgery. Scoliosis Research Society, 18th Annual Meeting, New Orleans, Louisiana, 1983.

4. Bonnett C, Brown JC, Perry J, Nichol VL, Walinski T, Brooks L, Hoffer M, Stiles C, Brooks R: Evolution of treatment of paralytic scoliosis at Rancho Los Amigos Hospital. J Bone Jt Surg 57A:206-215, 1975.

5. Luque ER: The anatomic basis and development of segmental spinal instrumentation. Spine 7:256-259, 1982.

6. MacEwen GD, Bunnell WP, Sriram K: Acute neurological complications in the treatment of scoliosis: a report of the Scoliosis Research Society. J Bone Jt Surg 57A:404-408, 1975.

7. Eismont FJ, Simeone FA: Bone overgrowth (hypertrophy) as a cause of late paraparesis after scoliosis fusion. J Bone Jt Surg 63A:1016-1019, 1981.

8. Liepeonis JV, Bunch WH, Lonser RE, Daley RM, Gogan UJ: Spinal cord injury during segmental sublamina spinal instrumentation: an animal model. Scoliosis Research Society, 18th Annual Meeting, New Orleans, Louisiana, 1983.

9. McAfee PC, Lubicky JP, Weiner FW: The use of segmental instrumentation to preserve longitudinal spinal growth. An experimental study. J Bone Jt Surg 65A:935-942, 1983.

10. Herring JA, Wenger DI: Segmental spinal instrumentation, preliminary report of 40 consecutive cases. Spine 7:285-298, 1982.

11. Gillespie R: Personal communication, 1983.

12. Nicastro JF, Traina J, Lancaster M, Hartgan C: Subliminal segmental wire fixation: anatomic pathways during their removal. Scoliosis Research Society, 18th Annual Meeting, New Orleans, Louisiana, 1983.

13. Wenger DR, Carollo JJ, Wilkerson JA: Biomechanics of scoliosis correction by segmental spinal instrumentation. Spine 7:260-264, 1982.

14. Letts RM, Hollenberg C: Delayed paresis following spine fusion with Harrington instrumentation. Clin Ortho Rel Res 125:45-48, 1977.

15. Eismont FJ, Wiesel SW, Rothman RH: Treatment of dural tears associated with spinal surgery. J Bone Jt Surg 63A:1132-1136, 1981.

16. Low TG: Segmental spinal instrumentation in the surgical treatment of Scheuermann's kyphosis. Scoliosis Research Society, 18th Annual Meeting, New Orleans, Louisiana, 1983.

17. McCarthy RE: A locking device for the Luque rods. Exhibit, Scoliosis Research Society, 18th Annual Meeting, New Orleans, Louisiana, 1983.

18. Guadagni T, Drummond D, Breed A: Strength of twisted stainless steel wire. Scoliosis Research Society, 18th Annual Meeting, New Orleans, Louisiana, 1983.

19. Mervyn-Evans E, Wales S, Freeman MAR, et al: Metal sensitivity as a cause of bone necrosis and loosening of the prosthesis in total joint replacement. J Bone Jt Surg 56B:626-642, 1974.

20. Kumar P, Bryan C, Bowler J, D'Ambrosia R, Leech SH, Mathews R: Metal hypersensitivity in total joint replacement. Orthopedics 6:1455-1458, 19

21. Luque ER: Personal communication, 1983.

22. Eberle CF: Early complications following Luque instrumentation in paralytic curves secondary to poliomyelitis. Scoliosis Research Society Meeting, Denver, 1982.

23. Taddonio RS: Segmental spinal instrumentation in the management of neuromuscular spinal deformity. Spine 7:305-311, 1982.

24. Herring JA, Wenger DR: Segmental spinal instrumentation: A preliminary report of 40 consecutive cases. Spine 7(3):285-298, 1982.

25. Luque ER: The anatomical basis and development of segmental spinal instrumentation. Spine 7(3):256-259, 1982.

26. Luque ER: Mistakes in segmental spinal instrumentation. Exhibit at Scoliosis Research Society, September, 1983.

27. Moe J, Denis F: The iatrogenic loss of lumbar lordosis. J Bone Jt Surg (Suppl) 1(2):131, 1977.

28. Sullivan AJ, Conner SB: Comparison of Harrington instrumentation and segmental spinal instrumentation in the management of neuromuscular spinal deformity. Spine 7(3):299-304, 1982.

29. Taddonio RF: Segmental spinal instrumentation in the management of neuromuscular spinal deformity. Spine 7(3):305-311, 1982.

INDEX